AF750732

Nutrition in care homes and home care

Report and recommendations: from recommendations to action

Committee of Experts on Nutrition, Food and Consumer Health (Partial Agreement) (P-SC-NU)

Council of Eur

19937531

The opinions expressed in this work are the responsibility of the authors and do not necessarily reflect the official policy of the Council of Europe.

All rights reserved. No part of this publication may be translated, reproduced or transmitted, in any form or by any means, electronic (CD-Rom, Internet, etc.) or mechanical, including photocopying, recording or any information storage or retrieval system, without prior permission in writing from the Public Information and Publications Division, Directorate of Communication (F-67075 Strasbourg Cedex or publishing@coe.int).

LIBRARY/DAWSON
PO-
Class No. 22Z COU
-2 FEB 2011
ce/Bar Code
Control No. a323888
19937531

Cover design: Graphic Design Workshop, Council of Europe

Council of Europe Publishing
F-67075 Strasbourg Cedex
http://book.coe.int

ISBN 978-92-871-6596-1
© Council of Europe, 2009
Printed in France

Table of contents

Table of figures

Preface

The Council of Europe

The Council of Europe is a political organisation which was founded on 5 May 1949 by 10 European countries in order to promote greater unity between its members. It now comprises 47 member states.[1]

The main aims of the Organisation are to reinforce democracy, human rights and the rule of law, and to develop common responses to political, social, cultural and legal challenges in its member states. Since 1989, the Council of Europe has integrated most of the countries of central and eastern Europe into its structures and supported them in their efforts to implement and consolidate their political, legal and administrative reforms.

The work of the Council of Europe has led, to date, to the adoption of over 200 European conventions and agreements, which create the basis for a common legal space in Europe. They include the European Convention on Human Rights (1950), the European Cultural Convention (1954), the European Social Charter (1961), the European Convention on the Prevention of Torture (1987) and the Convention on Human Rights and Bioethics (1997). Numerous recommendations and resolutions of the Committee of Ministers propose policy guidelines for national governments.

The Council of Europe has its permanent headquarters in Strasbourg (France). By statute, it has two constituent organs: the Committee of Ministers, composed of the Ministers for Foreign Affairs of the 47 member states, and the Parliamentary Assembly, comprising delegations from the 47 national parliaments. The Congress of Local and Regional Authorities of the Council of Europe represents the entities of local and regional self-government within the member states. A multinational European Secretariat serves these bodies and the intergovernmental committees.

The European Court of Human Rights is the judicial body competent to adjudicate complaints brought against a state by individuals, associations or other contracting states on grounds of violation of the European Convention on Human Rights.

---

1. Albania, Andorra, Armenia, Austria, Azerbaijan, Belgium, Bosnia and Herzegovina, Bulgaria, Croatia, Cyprus, Czech Republic, Denmark, Estonia, Finland, France, Georgia, Germany, Greece, Hungary, Iceland, Ireland, Italy, Latvia, Liechtenstein, Lithuania, Luxembourg, Malta, Moldova, Monaco, Montenegro, Netherlands, Norway, Poland, Portugal, Romania, Russian Federation, San Marino, Slovak Republic, Serbia, Slovenia, Spain, Sweden, Switzerland, "the former Yugoslav Republic of Macedonia", Turkey, Ukraine and the United Kingdom.

Partial Agreement in the Social and Public Health Field

When some, but not all, member states of the Council of Europe wish to engage in a certain activity, they can conclude a "Partial Agreement". The Partial Agreement in the Social and Public Health Field was concluded on this basis in 1959. It had 16 member states[2] before its dissolution on 31 December 2008.

Its areas of activity included the following two sectors:

- protection of public health;
- rehabilitation and integration of people with disabilities.

The above activities were entrusted to committees of experts that were answerable to one steering committee for each area. Close collaboration with other international institutions, in particular the Commission of the European Union was sought. Contact was also maintained with international non-governmental organisations (NGOs) and industry, working in similar or related fields.

Representatives of the European industry were entitled to attend meetings of ad hoc groups, which were advisory bodies to the committees of experts without the right to take formal decisions.

On specific questions, hearings were regularly organised between the committees of experts and the European industry.

The work of these committees occasionally results in the elaboration of conventions or agreements. The more usual outcome is the adoption, by the Committee of Ministers, of resolutions addressed to member states. Resolutions should be considered as statements of policy for national policy makers. Governments actively participate in their formulation and their delegates are usually both experts in the field in question and responsible for the implementation of government policy in their national ministries.

The procedure provides for considerable flexibility in that any state may reserve its position on a given point without thereby preventing the others from going ahead with what they consider appropriate. Another advantage is that the resolutions are readily susceptible to amendment should the need arise. Governments are furthermore called upon periodically to report on the implementation of the recommended measures.

2. Austria, Belgium, Cyprus, Denmark, Finland, France, Germany, Ireland, Netherlands, Norway, Portugal, Slovenia, Spain, Sweden, Switzerland and the United Kingdom.

A less formal procedure is the publication of general guidelines intended to serve as a model for member states.

Furthermore, scientific reports aimed at informing both governments and experts in the field are published on specific areas of concern.

Council of Europe committees in the field of nutrition, including compounds used in and on food

- Consumer Health Protection Committee (CD-P-SC) (steering committee, pursues activities of the former Public Health Committee);
- Committee of Experts on Nutrition, Food and Consumer Health (P-SC-NU)
- Committee of Experts on Materials Coming into Contact with Food (P-SC-CDA);
- ad hoc groups with specific focus and often with industry participation, such as coatings, cork, metals and alloys, paper and board, recycled fibres, packaging inks, ion exchange resins, rubber products and tissue papers;
- ad hoc groups of the Committee of Experts on Nutrition, Food and Consumer Health, with specific focus:
    - Ad hoc Group on Functional Food (with industry participation);
    - Ad hoc Group on Nutrition in Hospitals;
    - Ad hoc Group on Stored Product Protection;
- Committee of Experts on Flavouring Substances (P-SP-AR).

The present report and recommendations on nutrition in care homes and home care have been prepared by the Belgian delegation of the Committee of Experts on Nutrition, Food and Consumer Health (Partial Agreement) (P-SC-NU) and approved by the Council of Europe Consumer Health Protection Committee (Partial Agreement) (CD-P-SC).

For further information, please contact:

Council of Europe
F-67075 Strasbourg Cedex
France
Phone: +33 (0)3 88 41 20 00
Fax: +33 (0)3 88 41 27 81/82/83
Website: www.coe.int

Acknowledgements

This report was conceived in the framework of the Belgian National Food and Health Plan (NFHP-B) by M. Arvanitakis,[3] P. Coppens,[4] L. Doughan[5] and A. Van Gossum,[3] with the logistical and editorial support of C. Decroix.[6] The content is largely based on the recommendations and outcomes of the different working groups in the framework of the NFHP-B and the discussions, presentations and papers prepared by the speakers at the international workshop on undernutrition in care homes and home care, which was organised in Brussels on 22 and 23 November 2007 by the Belgian Federal Public Service of Health, Food Chain Safety and Environment.

The NFHP-B would like to thank:

– the speakers of the international workshop who reviewed this report and gave valuable comments: A. Beck,[7] F. De Man,[8] M. Elia,[9] X. Hebuterne,[10] S. Henry,[11] D.H. Jakobsen,[12] O. Kohl,[13] B. Lesourd,[14] H. Lochs,[15] H. Mostert,[16] T. Pepersack,[17] C. Pichard,[18] M. Planas,[19] K. Schindler,[20] J. Schols,[21] L. Sobotka[22] and J. Van Emelen;[23]

---

3. Nutrition Team, Erasme University Hospital, Brussels, Belgium.
4. European Advisory Services/National Food and Health Plan, Brussels, Belgium.
5. Federal Public Service of Health, Food Chain Safety and Environment/National Food and Health Plan, Brussels, Belgium.
6. Peak Communications, Brussels, Belgium.
7. National Food Institute, Technical University of Denmark, Copenhagen, Denmark.
8. The European Nutrition for Health Alliance, Brussels, Belgium.
9. Institute of Human Nutrition, University of Southampton, Southampton, UK.
10. Gastroenterology and Nutrition Clinic, CHU of Nice, Nice, France.
11. Ligue Nationale Alzheimer, Brussels, Belgium.
12. Unit of Perioperative Nursing, Copenhagen, Denmark.
13. Research and Development, Schubert Unternehmensgruppe GmbH, Düsseldorf, Germany.
14. Gerontology Department, Clermont-Ferrand University Hospital, Clermont-Ferrand, France.
15. Department of Gastroenterology, Hepatology and Endocrinology, Charité University Hospital, Berlin, Germany.
16. Vilans, Netherlands.
17. Geriatrics Department, Erasme University Hospital, Brussels, Belgium.
18. Clinical Nutrition Department, Geneva University Hospital, Geneva, Switzerland.
19. Nutritional Support Unit, General University Hospital Vall d'Hebron, Barcelona, Spain.
20. Department of Endocrinology, Vienna Medical Institute University, Vienna, Austria.
21. University of Maastricht and Vivre Care Group, Maastricht, Netherlands.

- the members of the various working groups of the NFHP-B who provided valuable input into this document: J.P. Baeyens, K. Boeykens, C. Corten, M. Delwaide, M. Declercq, R. De Donder, G. Dufourny, G. Filot, B. Folens, B. Geurden, M. Lardennois and R. Wouters;
- the members of the expert scientific group on undernutrition, which established the recommendations for screening and nutritional assessment annexed to this report: A. Van Gossum (president), I. Duysburgh, F. Mokaddem, T. Pepersack, S. Vereecken, I. Thiebaut, M. Declercq, M. Roosen, S. Martinuzzi, P. Milazzo, B. Geurden, K. Boeykens, R. Wauters, J. Damiaans, D. Dethier, P. Coppens, I. Laquiere and B. Folens;
- the members of the working group on care homes, which established the charter: K. Boeykens, C. Corten, C. Van Aelst, G. Filot, B. Folens, B. Geurden and P. Planche;
- the King Baudouin Foundation for their financial support;
- all the people who helped bring the topic of undernutrition into the spotlight and helped directly and indirectly to make this report possible.

22. Department of Metabolic Care and Gerontology, Medical Faculty of the Charles University, Hradec Kralove, Czech Republic.
23. Strategic Studies and Communication , Independent Health Insurance Funds, Brussels, Belgium.

Glossary

Anthropometrical measurements – Anthropometric assessment

The assessment of the nutritional state and body composition of a person. It may consist of measurements of height and body weight, skinfold thickness, and arm and calf circumferences.

Artificial nutritional support – Artificial feeding – Artificial nutrition

Administration of specially formulated liquid nutrients through a tube directly into the gut (enteral nutrition) or into a vein (parenteral nutrition).

Body Mass Index (BMI)

Weight (in kg) divided by height squared (in square metres). Used to define underweight, normal weight, overweight and obesity of adult people. However, people with low BMIs can be undernourished and oedema always falsely increases weight.

Caregiver – Carer

Unpaid relatives or friends whose life is in some way restricted by the need to be responsible for the care of someone who is mentally ill, mentally handicapped, physically disabled or whose health is impaired by sickness or old age.

Care home

Place of residence for people who require various degrees of constant nursing care because they have difficulties with the normal activities of daily living. Is also referred to as a nursing home, rest home or residential home. Residents can include old people or younger adults with physical disabilities.

Catabolic – Catabolism

The set of metabolic pathways that breakdown molecules into smaller units and release energy.

Clinical dietician

A dietician with an education in clinical nutrition and dietetics. Clinical dieticians are responsible for dietary prevention and treatment of individuals in institutions or the community.

Clinical nutrition

The application of scientifically based nutritional methods in medical practice. This includes nutritional prophylactics (disease prevention) as well as the treatment of nutritional disorders.

Comorbidity

The presence of one or more disorders (or diseases) in addition to a primary disease or disorder

Community dietician

Community dieticians carry out clinical-based patient care in the form of home visits for patients who are too physically ill to attend a consultation in health facilities.

Complex carbohydrates

Refers to carbohydrate sources rich in dietary fibre, such as fruit, vegetables and whole grains.

Cost-benefit

The analysis extends the cost-effectiveness analysis by placing a monetary value on the outcomes.

Cost-effectiveness

Compares two or more different ways to achieve the same objective.

Council of residents

Committee composed of representatives of the residents in care homes.

Disease-related undernutrition

A state of insufficient intake, utilisation or absorption of energy and nutrients due to individual or systemic factors, which results in recent or rapid weight loss and change in organ function, and is likely to be associated with a worse outcome from the disease or the treatment. Undernourished people can be overweight or obese according to their BMI.

Energy- and protein-dense menu

A menu with a high nutrient density, due to the use of food products with a high fat and protein content.

Enteral nutrition

Nutrition provided through a tube, catheter or stoma that delivers nutrients distal to the oral cavity.

First-line health care workers

The health care workers who are involved with primary care. They act as a first point of consultation for the patients. They provide the widest scope of health care, including for patients of all ages. Continuity is also a key characteristic of care provided by primary care workers (also referred to as front-line health care workers).

Food service – Meals-on-wheels – Catering service

A system in which meals are produced and served for people residing in health care facilities (hospitals, care homes), in a professional context. The system includes the food service premises, the production and distribution technology, and human resources involved in management, production, distribution and serving.

General dietician

A dietician with an education in clinical nutrition and dietetics, and food service management with overall responsibility for both aspects in an institution or a community.

General practitioner – Family doctor – Physician

Medical practitioner who provides primary care and specialises in family medicine.

Global medical record – Medical record – Health record

Refers to a systematic documentation of a person's medical care and history. The term "medical record" is used both for the physical folder for each individual patient and for the body of information that comprises each patient's health history.

Health care worker – Health care professionals

All "professional caregivers", including general physicians, nurses, dieticians, speech therapists, physiotherapists, pharmacists, etc., who are paid to deliver care to patients and old people. Unlike caregivers who provide care on a voluntary basis, they are normally paid.

Home care

Health care or supportive care provided in a person's home by health care professionals and caregivers.

Inpatient

A patient who occupies a hospital bed.

Institution

Any health care facility where people are admitted for acute or chronic care, typically including hospitals and nursing or care homes.

Macronutrients

Energy-supplying nutrients (carbohydrates, proteins, and lipids).

Malnutrition

A deficiency or excess of energy, protein and other nutrients causing adverse effects on tissue, body form (body shape, size and composition) and function, as well as on clinical outcomes.

Malnutrition Universal Screening Tool (MUST)

Screening tool for undernutrition, developed by BAPEN (2004). Recommended by the NFHP-B as a reference tool in geriatric hospital patients (>75 years) and in younger people in home care settings.

Metabolic rate

the rate of energy expended while at rest in a neutrally temperate environment, in the post-absorptive state (meaning that the digestive system is inactive).

Micronutrients

Essential nutrients present and required in the body in small quantities (vitamins, minerals and oligoelements).

Mini Nutritional Assessment (MNA)

Screening tool for undernutrition, developed by Nestlé Nutrition Services (1998). Recommended by the NFHP-B as a reference tool in care homes and in geriatric hospital patients (>75 years). The short form of the MNA (questions A to F – MNA-SF) is the preferred method for screening in the home care situation.

Nursing home

See "care home".

Nutrition charter

Charter explicating requirements to be met for accreditation in relation to nutritional care (see appendix).

Nutrition committee – Nutritional support team

Multidisciplinary team in an institution in charge of the development and implementation of nutritional screening, assessment and support protocols.

Nutrition manager

The person in charge of the nutrition committee, usually a specialist doctor with expertise in nutrition.

Nutritional assessment

A comprehensive evaluation of nutritional status, including one or more of the following: medical history, dietary history, physical examination, anthropometrical measurements and laboratory data.

Nutritional care

The basic duty of providing adequate and appropriate food and drinks, and/or artificial nutrition to a person.

Nutritional patient record

Systematic documentation of a person's nutritional care and history, either in physical form (nutrition status booklet, etc.) or electronically. Should be part of the global medical record of the person.

Nutritional risk

The risk for nutrition-related complications to the disease or the treatment.

Nutritional risk screening (NRS-2002)

The process of identifying characteristics known to be associated with nutrition-related complications. Its purpose is to detect persons at risk who may experience an improved clinical outcome when given nutritional support.

The term is also used to describe a screening tool for undernutrition, developed by an ad hoc ESPEN working group (2002). This tool is recommended by the NFHP-B as a reference tool in general hospital patients.

Nutritional steering committee

An advisory committee consisting of staff from all disciplines, including managers, involved in the nutritional care of the patient or resident in the institution.

Nutritional support

Assessment of current nutritional status, estimation of nutritional requirements, prescription and delivery of appropriate energy, macro- and micronutrients, electrolytes and fluids (in the form of ordinary hospital food (first choice), sip feedings and/or artificial nutrition), monitoring the former in the context of clinical status and ensuring that the most optimal feeding route is used at all times. Nutritional support is part of the medical treatment and its purpose is to improve or maintain a person's nutritional status and hasten and improve recovery.

Nutritional support teams/units (NST)

A multidisciplinary team/unit with expertise in nutrition, which is involved in nutritional support and the remit of which varies according to local circumstances, interest and resource allocation. Usually takes active part in nutritional support, and serves in a quality control capacity, standardising practice, gathering new information and educating other health care professionals.

Outpatient

A patient who comes to the hospital, clinic, or dispensary for diagnosis and/or treatment but does not occupy a bed.

Parenteral nutrition

Nutrients provided intravenously either into a large central vein or a peripheral vein.

Patient

A person requiring medical treatment, either staying at the hospital (inpatient), visiting the hospital without occupying a bed (outpatient) or being treated by a general practitioner.

Reimbursement

Full or partial compensation given by the state to a person for an expense (for example, when dietician consultation or the use of supplemental foods is indicated, reimbursement could help avoid financial barriers).

Resident

A person staying at a care home.

Sarcopenia

The degenerative loss of skeletal muscle mass, strength and integrity associated with senescence (advanced age).

Sip feeding

The oral administration of nutritional support under the form of supplemental feeds (most frequently under the form of drinks).

Stakeholders – Society stakeholders

Any person, institution or organisation that has an interest in a certain topic.

Subjective Global Assessment (SGA)

Nutritional assessment method, described by Detsky, Mclaughin and Baker (1987). It assesses nutritional status based on features of the history and physical examination. This tool is recommended by the NFHP-B as a reference tool for nutritional assessment in all settings (hospital, care home, home care).

Supplements – Supplemental foods – Supplemental feeds

Foodstuffs that are specifically formulated (enriched in energy, protein and/or vitamins and minerals) to provide appropriate nutritional support in specific diseases and/or (disease-related) undernutrition. When produced by companies, they are legally called foods for special medical purposes. Compositional and other aspects are regulated at EU level by Directive 1999/21.

Tube feeding – Enteral feeding

The administration of nutritional support under the form of supplemental feeds by using a feeding tube inserted into the gastrointestinal tract. It is either nasogastric (down the oesophagus into the stomach) or gastric (through a small incision in the abdomen into the stomach, most frequently by percutaneous gastric endoscopy).

Undernutrition

A condition that is characterised by clinical depletion, undesired weight loss or underweight.

Wasting

The process by which muscle and fat tissue “wastes” away, caused by low food intake or debilitating diseases.

Abbreviations

AIM: Association Internationale de la Mutualité

BAPEN: British Association of Parenteral and Enteral Nutrition

BMI = Body Mass Index (expressed as kg/m^2 ($weight/height^2$))

DGE: German Nutrition Society

DGEM: German Society for Nutritional Medicine

EN: enteral nutrition

ENDA: European Nursing Directors Association

ESPEN: European Society for Clinical Nutrition and Metabolism

EUGMS: European Union Geriatric Medicine Society

FENS: Federation of European Nutrition Societies

FTE: full-time equivalent

GP: general practitioner

HACCP: hazard analysis critical control points

HOPE: European Hospital and Healthcare Federation

ILC: International Longevity Centre-UK

LPZ: Landelijke Prevalentiemeting Zorgproblemen project

MNA: Mini Nutritional Assessment

MNA-SF: Mini Nutritional Assessment Short Form

MNI: Medical Nutrition International Industry

MUST: Malnutrition Universal Screening Tool

NCPC: National Council for Palliative Care

NFHP-B: Belgian National Food and Health Plan

ONS: oral nutritional supplements

PCM: protein calorie malnutrition

PEM: protein energy malnutrition

RDA: recommended daily allowance

SGA: Subjective Global Assessment

TPN: total parenteral nutrition

Executive summary

Undernutrition is a deficiency of energy, protein and other nutrients impairing the body and its functioning, jeopardising clinical outcomes. Undernutrition causes hospital stays to double and increases complications and mortality with the elderly across Europe. Among the causes of undernutrition are decreased metabolic rate, weaknesses and illnesses. Complicating factors common with the elderly are loss of appetite, dementia, social isolation, reduced oral health, financial problems and absence of feeding assistance – making this group particularly vulnerable to undernutrition.

Treating undernutrition costs around €10.95 billion per year in the case of the UK, thus making it as costly as, for example, obesity. Although most of the expenditure on disease-related malnutrition involves people over 65, or 15% of the population, it remains largely unrecognised as a major health care problem. About half the cost of undernutrition occurs outside hospitals, mainly in long-term residential care for older people. Care costs can be reduced through preventive medicine, observing social justice and fair equity-efficiency trade-offs. Undernutrition can be prevented through promoting better nutrition in hospitals and care homes and oral hygiene, by installing screening routines, by educating caregivers, and by making meals a social event. Reimbursement should be expanded for dietary counselling and supplemental foods.

Proper screening routines are of particular importance for early detection of undernutrition, which can be concealed. Health care facilities need to adopt scientifically and technically established diagnosis tools and criteria, and should continue screening after discharge from hospital. Collaboration with dieticians should be increased. To successfully tackle malnutrition a multidisciplinary, multilevel approach is important, informing, educating and training stakeholders, patients and residents, family, caregivers and policy makers. Awareness of undernutrition issues should be improved with care home management and kitchen staff through continued education. Dieticians should be given a central role in this regard. In the light of the above, policy makers should create legal frameworks to confront undernutrition as the public health concern that it is. Governments should set and enforce standards for nutritional care and screening, assessment and follow-up and make undernutrition part of national food and health plans. Dietetic follow-up and specialised nutrition should be included for reimbursement. Support should be given to research on best practices, and evidence-based approaches. National platforms for the transfer of nutritional patient information between care settings should be organised. Nutritional education should be included in physicians', nurses' and caregivers' training. Finally, government policies aimed at combating undernutrition should include assigning political responsibility for elderly people and putting undernutrition on the political agenda.

1. Introduction

In 2002, the Council of Europe published a report on food and nutritional care in hospitals,[i] which contained over 100 recommendations for improvement. In this report, the Council of Europe confirms that early and proactive screening, combined with the monitoring of dietary habits, can contribute to a faster socio-economic reintegration of the patient and to an improvement of his/her quality of life. In 2003, the Council of Europe Committee of ministers adopted a resolution[ii] and formulated recommendations on the situation in hospitals. These recommendations include:

- a clear definition of the responsibilities of health care staff and hospital management with regard to nutritional care;
- implementation of scientific standards for assessing, evaluating and supervising diet and the risks of patients in relation to undernutrition;
- extension of an institution's liability with regards to nutritional care after hospitalisation;
- improving the training level of health care staff;
- promotion of individualised and flexible offer of meals with the possibility for the patient to ask for additional servings;
- patients' input into drafting their meal-taking schedule;
- promotion of co-operation and communication amongst hospital staff members to guarantee an optimal level of nutritional care, including better communication between the hospital and front-line health care staff;
- the notion that far from being a hotel service, nutrition is an essential element of patient treatment; it must therefore be considered as such by the hospital management;
- the idea that management must acknowledge responsibility for dispensing nutritional care and must give priority to an internal policy on nutrition;
- taking into account the costs incurred by complications and prolongation of hospital stays due to undernutrition when allocating the food budget.

In 2006, as an example of national activities, the Belgian National Food and Health Plan[iii] was initiated to address nutritional and health issues and formulate related recommendations. It focuses on three different settings: hospitals, care homes and home care. The plan considered undernutrition as an important issue, which led to the establishment of a dedicated policy option and the creation of several expert working groups. Their main objective was to identify the main causes of undernutrition and develop an action plan. This resulted in the identification of eight fields of action. A two-day international workshop on the topic of undernutrition in care homes and home care was organised on 22 and 23 November 2007 and allowed European experts to present and debate the various aspects of this specific problem in Europe.

These activities together with the Council of Europe Committee of Ministers resolution have been the basis for the recommendations and evaluations in this report. It focuses on the importance of early and adequate nutritional risk screening, the prevalence and causes of undernutrition, the different types of nutritional support, the distribution of responsibilities and the importance of continuing education on (clinical) nutrition in the three settings. At the end of this report, we will outline the responsibilities of all the actors involved in resolving this important European-wide issue, as well as suggesting possible actions in each of the settings.

The following have served as sources of information for this report:

- the report and recommendations of the Committee of Experts on Nutrition, Food Safety and Consumer Protection, *Food and nutritional care in hospitals: how to prevent undernutrition*, 2003;
- papers and the report prepared by speakers at the international workshop on undernutrition in care homes and home care, Brussels, November 2007;[iv]
- the recommendations and outcomes of the different working groups in the framework of the Belgian National Food and Health Plan (NFHP-B), 2006-08;[iii]
- the final report of the STAVO project conducted by the Belgian Ministry of Social Affairs and Public Health, 2006;[v]
- the evaluation report of a project on undernutrition in geriatric wards, conducted by the Belgian Ministry of Social Affairs and Public Health, 2007.[vi]

2. Prevalence and causes of undernutrition in care homes and home care

Summary

- the diagnosis of severe undernutrition is based on the presence of one or more of the following criteria: (1) weight loss ≥ 10% in one month or ≥ 15% in six months; (2) BMI < 18 kg/m^2; (3) serum albumin < 30 g/l;
- undernutrition is frequent in older individuals living at home (8-19%) and in chronic care institutions (26-38%) according to various European prevalence studies;
- older people are at risk of micronutrient deficiency (mainly group B vitamins, vitamin C, vitamin D, selenium, zinc and calcium).
- causes that lead to undernutrition include oral and dental disorders, swallowing problems, depression, dementia, chronic diseases, medication, and psychological and social factors leading to dependency.

Undernutrition

Although specific numbers are scarce, there is a consensus amongst various stakeholders that undernutrition remains a considerable problem in health care settings and policies all over Europe. Undernutrition is usually defined as a deficiency or excess of energy, protein and other nutrients causing adverse effects on tissue, body form (body shape, size and composition) and function, as well as on clinical outcomes.[vii] This report focuses specifically on undernutrition, a condition which is characterised by clinical depletion, undesired weight loss or underweight. Sometimes, undernutrition is also defined by the terms protein calorie malnutrition (PCM), protein energy malnutrition (PEM) or malnutrition of multiple nutrients. The condition results from an imbalance between intake and bodily requirements. This imbalance causes tissue loss, in particular of muscle tissue, with harmful functional consequences.

Nutrition deficits result in major body dysfunctions altering daily activities (autonomy), increasing the prevalence of additional pathologies (vulnerability) and delaying recovery after acute events (clinical outcome), and ultimately jeopardising the economic system of the health care institutions.

Poor nutritional intake, physical inactivity, chronic diseases and ageing pave the way for undernutrition. These conditions are generally not recognised as "risk situations" and are therefore not medically taken into account in due time in order to allow optimal treatment, such as timely nutritional support. At later stages, severe undernutrition is difficult and costly to cure.

As prevention is both easier and more cost-effective, screening for the risk of undernutrition is therefore a first important public health measure to identify people at risk.

In guidelines established in France in 2007 by the Haute Autorité de Santé, the risk of undernutrition is defined by the presence of at least one of the following criteria:[viii]

- weight loss ≥ 5% over one month or ≥ 10% over six months;
- Body Mass Index (BMI) < 21 kg/m^2;
- serum albumin concentrations < 35 g/l;
- Global Mini Nutritional Assessment (MNA) score < 17.

If these criteria are met, a person will have an increased risk of actually developing undernutrition if appropriate action is not taken. The diagnosis of severe undernutrition is based on the presence of one or more of the following criteria:

- weight loss ≥ 10% in one month or ≥ 15% in six months;
- BMI < 18 kg/m^2;
- serum albumin < 30 g/l.

Prevalence

There is a general agreement that undernutrition in Europe is significant, especially among older people (20-30% for BMI < 20 kg/m^2). The Council of Europe, in its 2003 resolution on food and nutritional care in hospitals, even went as far as saying that there is an "unacceptable number of undernourished hospital patients in Europe". It is also important to state that the risk of undernutrition increases during hospital stays.

It is very difficult to assess the prevalence of undernutrition in both care homes and home care, and to compare various figures between different countries, since there is as yet no general agreement on the criteria that should be used when establishing the prevalence of undernutrition in adults (including old people). Different methods and criteria have been used and have led to a broad variety of figures on prevalence, but it is important to assess a person's nutritional status with proper and user-friendly methods, such as weight loss, BMI, (recent) food intake, age-related changes in body composition, muscle mass and function, etc.[ix]

Some countries, like the Netherlands, have a set of clear measurement and screening tools, but there is an obvious need for a tool that is agreed on and used by all European countries. Studies should therefore be undertaken to develop and validate simple screening methods for examining undernutrition in care homes and home care. In Chapter 6 of this report, some possible screening methods are listed, together with the issues currently related to the screening of undernutrition.

Nursing homes

In Belgium, a survey on the prevalence of undernutrition in geriatric wards of 90 hospitals showed that four out of five people suffer from undernutrition or are at risk. Out of the 2 565 people aged 75 and older who were admitted to a geriatric ward, 35.9% suffered from undernutrition and 41.9% were found to be at risk using their MNA score.[vi]

Figures from France estimate that undernutrition affects between 4% and 10% of older people living at home; 15-38% of those in institutional care; and 30-70% of hospitalised older people. A study aimed at describing the nutritional status of geriatric home residents according to their place of dwelling in the Aquitaine region estimated the prevalence of undernutrition to be 19.1%. This rate was higher in long-term care (48.0%) than in nursing homes (14.5%).[x]

The prevalence of undernutrition at home (8-12%) shows that we need to prevent undernutrition in the general population. Its prevalence at the time of hospital admission (30-50%, higher in geriatrics) indicates the vulnerability of undernourished people. During hospitalisation, undernutrition is an aggravating factor in the main because pre-existing undernutrition is not recognised, food intake is chronically insufficient and nutritional support, if prescribed, is too late to be efficient.

In the Netherlands, a National Prevalence Measurement of Care Problems is conducted annually (since 1998) in home care organisations, care homes and hospitals (LPZ project).[xi] It provides insight into the prevalence, prevention, management and quality indicators of relevant care problems. It is a cross-sectional study with a standardised questionnaire, carried out one day a year (four days in home care), during which all persons are assessed by two caregivers per person (for assessment). Since 2004, the prevalence and other indicators of undernutrition are also measured annually. The LPZ project uses the following definition to identify undernutrition:

- BMI < 18.5 kg/m^2 (< 24 kg/m^2 if age ≥ 85);
- or unintentional weight loss (6 kg during last six months or 3 kg during the last month);
- or a BMI between 18.5 and 20 kg/m^2 (24-29 kg/m^2 if age ≥ 85) in combination with no nutritional intake for three days or likelihood of less intake for more than one week.

In this study, involving 12 883 people, the prevalence was shown to be the highest in hospitals (23.8%) followed by home care organisations (21.7%) and nursing homes (19.2%).[xii] The evolution of the prevalence of undernutrition in the Netherlands during the period 2004-07 is shown below in Figure 1.[xiii]

Malnutrition (%)				
Organisation	2004	2005	2006	2007
Acute care				
Academic hospitals	26.0	29.7	29.9	16.5
General hospitals	28.2	26.5	23.3	16.1
Chronic care				
Nursing homes	24.0	20.7	25.6	22.3
Residential homes	18.5	17.9	28.0	26.2
Home care				
Home care organisation	28.7	24.9	22.9	19.3

Figure 1: Prevalence of undernutrition in the Netherlands 2004-07[24]

24. "Landelijke Prevalentiemeting Zorgproblemen. Rapportage resultaten. 2007", www.lpz-um.nl/documents/lpz/lpz_rapport_2007_secured.pdf, p. 15. Date of consultation: 27 October 2008.

Home care

In Belgium, a survey – the NAME study, 1997[xiv] – of people aged over 60 illustrates that undernutrition is also of concern in the home care setting. Nutritional assessment using MNA showed that 45% of this population group had an increased risk of undernutrition and that undernutrition was present in 6%.

Amongst the factors that have a negative influence on nutritional status, the survey showed that of the people in the survey:

- 50% were completely dependent on others for the preparation of the main hot meal;
- 17% were dependent on hot meal delivery services;
- 36% do not always finish their meal;
- 14% seldom or never enjoy their meals;
- 73% have orthodontic prostheses and 10% do not wear them during eating;
- 30% do not have a food shop in their neighbourhood or cannot reach it;
- 10% have frequent financial problems; in 3% these problems are serious.

Causes

Risk of undernutrition increases with age. In all health care settings, including care homes and home care, the percentage of people suffering from undernutrition rises when the number of diseases as well as care dependency increases.

Obviously, the most important cause of undernutrition is reduced or insufficient intake of food or increased loss of nutrients. In older people in particular, the process of ageing induces physiological and behavioural changes that negatively affect nutritional intake. Weakness and associated illnesses, loss of appetite, dental problems, lack of help with eating, social isolation, financial problems, etc., are all factors leading to reduced food intake. Moreover, many diseases have anorexia as a symptom, which in itself may lead to undernutrition.[xv]

Furthermore, many frequently occurring conditions in older people are also known to affect adequate nutritional intake indirectly. Conditions leading to memory loss, such as dementia or Alzheimer's disease, impair communication skills and result in a loss of autonomy with regard to food choice and eating. Ultimately, it makes the person completely dependent on the care of others. People gradually lose their taste perception and food preferences, which lead to decreased food intake. The rhythm of feeding changes, with excessive intake or lack of intake at moments and unbalanced intake because of limited or monotonous food preferences. Although not the only factor, reduced food intake invariably results in wasting and considerable loss of weight in people at the advanced stage of the disease. Mobility becomes a serious problem and the risk of aspiration of food, leading to pneumonia, increases.

Emotional problems are one of the most common reversible causes of undernutrition, particularly in old people. As already mentioned, financial problems are another important factor for 10% of older people. Because of their social isolation, financial problems, etc., older people frequently lose their lust for life and food and reduce their food intake. This loss of "appetite for life" is aggravated by disease, disabilities (difficulties in swallowing, chewing, oral pain, etc.) and medication. This situation can result in long periods of insufficient energy intake and loss of weight. Emotional problems as a consequence of the prior illness, social isolation or bereavement can easily lead to apathy and anorexia, causing undernutrition and possibly creating a vicious cycle. Undernutrition, in combination with the underlying disorder, increases the risk of complications, lowers resistance to infections, impairs wound healing, harms the person's physical and emotional condition still more and is likely to increase the risk of mortality.[xvi]

Avoiding isolation, developing adapted housing and allowing old people to take their meal in a family environment rather than isolated meal services are elements that can reduce emotional factors leading to undernutrition. Housing that favours social interaction between young and old, development of autonomy and opening up to the exterior world do exist, in amongst other countries Denmark, Netherlands and Canada, but also in Belgium (group housing like the beguine convents, the Abbeyfield houses, host families, kangaroo housing, housing shared with a student and bi-generational housing). It has been shown that family-style meals stimulate daily energy intake and protect nursing home residents against undernutrition.[xvii]

It is therefore important to recognise risk factors that may be present. Such risk factors for undernutrition in older people include factors unrelated to age and factors more specific to older people. The main risk factors unrelated to age are cancer, chronic and severe organ failure (cardiac, respiratory, renal or hepatic), gastrointestinal diseases causing indigestion and/or malabsorption, chronic alcoholism, chronic infectious and/or inflammatory diseases, progressive neurological diseases and all factors likely to cause a reduction in food intake, an increase in energy requirements, malabsorption, or all three. An overview of the most common risk factors in relation to the development of undernutrition is given below in Figure 2.[xviii]

Factor	Possible causes
Psychological, social and environmental	Social isolation Grieving Financial difficulties Ill-treatment Hospitalisation Change in lifestyle: admission to an institution
Oral and dental disorders	Mastication disorders Poor dental status Poorly fitting dentures Dryness of the mouth Oropharyngeal candidiasis Dysgueusia
Swallowing disorders	ENT disease* Vascular neurodegenerative disease
Psychiatric disorders	Depressive syndromes Behavioural disorders
Dementia	Alzheimer's disease Other forms of dementia
Other neurological disorders	Confusional syndrome Consciousness disorders Parkinsonism

* Diseases of the ear, nose and throat

Factor	Possible causes
Long-term drug treatment	Polymedication Medication causing dryness of the mouth, dysgueusia, gastrointestinal disorders, anorexia, drowsiness, etc. Long-term corticosteroid therapy
Any acute disorder or decompensation of a chronic disease	Pain Infectious disease Fracture causing a disability Surgical procedure Severe constipation Pressure sores
Dependency for daily activities	Eating dependency Mobility dependency
Restrictive diets	Salt-free Slimming Diabetic Cholesterol-lowering Long-term residue-free diets

Figure 2: Risk factors in relation to the development of undernutrition[25]

25. Haute Authorité de Santé, "Clinical Practice Guidelines. Nutritional support strategy for protein-energy malnutrition in the elderly", April 2007, www.has-

Each of these factors may promote or be associated with undernutrition and must alert the health professionals and close relatives to an increased risk. This is especially the case if several factors are combined.

Lack of awareness is a crucial factor in the persistence of undernutrition. A Dutch study, carried out by TNS-NIPO in 2000, reported that 60-80% of general practitioners do not experience undernutrition as a problem in their practice.[xix] In hospitals and care homes, professionals do not realise that undernutrition is so prevalent and is often already present on admission. In home care there is even less attention paid to this problem.

In the home care setting, the main contributing factors to the risk of undernutrition are therefore the lack of awareness and the difficulty to screen and assess people in the home environment. Paramedical professionals and caregivers often have limited resources and time and are focused on care-related aspects rather than on nutrition. Lack of communication with the person's physician and lack of awareness of undernutrition add to the problem. When people are immobilised or incapacitated, or when they have financial problems, proper nutrition is often the first element that is neglected.

Many older people living in care homes or at home are bound to go to a hospital at a given moment because of various illnesses. When such people are at risk or already suffering from undernutrition, such a hospital stay is often deleterious for their nutritional status. Not only will these people already be suffering from loss of appetite caused by their disease and medication, but the diagnostic and (surgical) interventions in the hospital will often result in a diminished digestion and/or intake of important nutritional elements. Most people have an energy and protein intake below the estimated requirements, and an accordingly low intake and blood level of vitamins and minerals.[xx] This problem is aggravated due to a lack of systematic screening and nutritional care, a lack of education and training of the caregivers, and an absence of criteria and quality standards for the food offered to the people (inappropriate dietary choice, interruption of meals by the staff, missed meals due to different procedures, etc.).

---

sante.fr/portail/upload/docs/application/pdf/malnutrition_elderly_guidelines.pdf, p. 8. Date of consultation: 27 October 2008.

Specific recommendations with regard to prevalence and causes:

- promote better nutrition offering/oral hygiene;
- avoid social isolation;
- include best practices for screening and nutritional assessment in the education and training of primary health workers;
- raise the awareness of health workers through systematic training to enable them to recognise undernutrition at an early stage and to start appropriate treatment;
- deploy a systematic screening of residents, at the level of care homes;
- raise the awareness of first-line care in order to screen people who live at home, to struggle against social isolation and to develop housing policies that are especially adapted;
- develop strategies that allow older people to realise their wishes, namely by rethinking the architecture of the proposed housing to promote social interaction and avoid isolation;
- replace meal services with family-style meals in nursing homes so as to make it possible to take a meal in a family style in the canteens of nursing homes;
- pay special attention to the particular situation of the nutritional intake of people aged 85 and over and people with chronic diseases.

3. Consequences of undernutrition for older people

Summary

- undernutrition may prolong the patient's hospital stay, increase the rate of complications by up to 20 times and increase death rates compared to well-nourished patients with the same diseases;
- sarcopenia with muscle wasting is also a consequence of undernutrition, which may lead to respiratory failure and physical dependency;
- undernutrition can lead to a state of social isolation and high level of dependence.

Morbidity – Mortality

The number of older people is constantly rising, especially in European countries and North America. These people also constitute a growing group of people who are admitted to hospitals due to acute or chronic illness. However, combinations of numerous chronic diseases with lack of functional ability make this group very vulnerable; Their treatment is more complicated and expensive and the results are uncertain. Moreover, severe protein energy undernutrition has been found in 26-65% of older hospital in-patients and in 5-85% of institutionalised individuals. The loss of lean body mass is frequently connected with this poor outcome. A clear relationship is found between mortality and nutritional status, assessed anthropometrically in hip fracture patients.[xxi,xxii,xxiii,xxiv]

As stated in Chapter 3, undernutrition increases the risk of complications, and severely undernourished patients often enter a cycle of progressive clinical deterioration. Their hospital stay may be twice as long as normal, and complications and death rates may be 20 times higher than well-nourished patients with the same diseases.[xxv] Because they do not take in the necessary vitamins and food elements, they are – because of their nutritional deficits – often unable to recover from the first condition whilst developing a second. They also suffer from impaired resistance to infection, which in turn can worsen their nutritional status.

Another consequence of undernutrition in older people is loss of muscle mass (sarcopenia), which is not only a consequence of poor nutrition but is also the result of complex factors such as immobility, ongoing chronic diseases, hormonal changes, oxidative stress, etc. Immobility in particular can play an important role in its development. The loss of muscle mass contributes to limitations in physical activity and decreases the capacity for rehabilitation especially in older patients. Then even a small decrease in muscle mass (which occurs during acute illness) significantly decreases the capacity for the basic activities mentioned above. Whereas in young and previously healthy people the loss of muscle mass only decreases their capability for certain extra activities (sport, climbing the stairs, running, etc.), the loss of muscle mass in older "depleted" patients leads to the loss of very basic activities. This leads to their dependency and can even cause significant problems with keeping an upright position and coughing.

The amount of muscle tissue is closely related to physical activity; however, physical activity among the elderly is frequently reduced to events like going to the bathroom, washing, taking meals and sometimes also food preparation or a short walk outside the apartment. Undoubtedly, decreased muscle function as a result of insufficient physical activity (because of age or disease) is a factor that contributes to further loss of muscle tissue. Furthermore, sarcopenia, aggravated by undernutrition, increases the risk of a fall, a leading cause for admission to hospital of older people. In the presence of undernutrition and/or sarcopenia, recovery from fractures is greatly impaired, resulting in increased morbidity and mortality.

Acute diseases such as inflammation as well as surgery or trauma lead to further muscle wasting. Muscle protein catabolism accelerates to balance substrate demands for tissue repair and gluconeogenesis. These substrates are necessary for survival but in extreme cases catabolic response can result in such dysfunction and tissue loss that survival is threatened even in young subjects. There is a reduced amount of substrate, which fluxes between muscles and injured tissues (trauma, operation wound, bedsores, site of inflammation, etc.), and this decreases the inflammatory, immune and healing processes in older patients with prior undernutrition. Probably all these mechanisms are responsible for the higher mortality rate apparent in people who are undernourished or at risk of undernutrition.

Particular attention should be paid to a loss of mass of the respiratory muscles, which makes it difficult for the older person to cough and expectorate effectively, with an increased risk of lung infection as a result. Multiple aspirations and fatal pneumonia are frequent consequences of such a development. An impaired ventilatory drive may also make it difficult to take a critically ill patient off the ventilator. The cardiac function is impaired, with a reduced cardiac output and a risk of heart failure. Gastrointestinal function and structure are impaired. Loss of mobility as a consequence of reduced muscle mass not only delays recovery, but also predisposes the patient to thromboembolism and bedsores.

Even older people who survive acute illness treatment are for a long time fully dependent on the help of others and quite often spend the rest of their lives in care homes. The resulting dependence further deteriorates the mental state of already catabolic patients. This leads to profound depression, anorexia and to the fixation of the futile cycle described above. In this way, older people who were mentally relatively stable before their acute illness will face substantial psychological and physical problems during several days after acute illness or elective surgery. Unfortunately, this change is often misinterpreted as a mental impairment and treatment with neuroleptic drugs frequently terminates the patient's life.

A rapid weight loss of between 5% and 10% causes clinically significant changes in organ functions; a weight loss between 35% and 40% is associated with a 30% risk of death, and survival beyond 50% weight loss is unlikely.

At its worst, undernutrition leads to death, either from a preventable complication or from inanition. The sequence of anorexia of the ageing leading to sarcopenia, leading to cachexia is the futile cycle that has to be broken by early screening and appropriate treatment.

Quality of life

It is clear that all of the above-mentioned consequences ultimately result in a decreased "quality of life" for the undernourished older person.

As described above, undernutrition results in increased immobility and dependency on others. Undernutrition limits the physical activities, and even severely decreases the capacity of performing basic activities for these older people. This in turn leads to a loss of autonomy, a decrease in social interactions, and further isolation and alienation, thus aggravating undernutrition.

Undernutrition makes the person become apathetic and depressed, which may lead to a loss of morale and the will to recover. The inability to concentrate also means that the person cannot benefit from instructions about techniques needed for self-care. A general sense of weakness impairs the appetite and the ability to eat.

Undernutrition clearly leads to a state of social isolation and a high level of dependence.

Good nutrition is a synonym of health-related quality of life. It averts undernutrition, prevents dietary deficiency disease and promotes optimal functioning. Because of its consequences on both physical and mental health, undernutrition severely affects the quality of life of people affected by it.

Specific recommendations with regard to the consequences of undernutrition for older people:

- develop social policies that favour social interaction among generations and structures that allow older people to stay in their homes, by financing adapted housing and by offering catering services of high nutritional quality.

4. Impact of undernutrition on health care costs

Summary

- undernutrition-related disease is an economic burden in most countries and preventive medicine should therefore be one of the cornerstones of actions undertaken to reduce health care costs;
- cost-effectiveness analysis, which should take into account social justice and an appropriate equity-efficiency trade-off, is important to determine appropriate management;
- hospital-related undernutrition and its costs could be reduced by better general hospital food provision and medical reimbursement, including that for artificial nutrition, as well as a smooth transition between hospital and chronic care centres.

Optimal nutrition and dietary goals in older people

Dietary factors are the most preventable cause of illness. As the main providers of health care in Europe, health care facilities are expected to serve nutritious, tasty meals that support and stimulate recovery from illness, and promote a healthy, balanced diet. Unfortunately, several surveys and official reports have shown the dissatisfaction of hospital patients and care home residents with the food offered. Regulators are therefore concerned that the health of patients is being undermined, leading to longer hospital stays and in consequence unnecessary and avoidable costs to health care.

In general, at an international level, health care costs are continuously increasing. Preventive public health, however, only accounts for 0.5-6% of all health care costs, which is clearly insufficient.

It is a general observation that the costs of health care, having risen considerably in the past decade, continue to rise. This is an observation valid for all EU countries (see Figure 3 below).[xxvi]

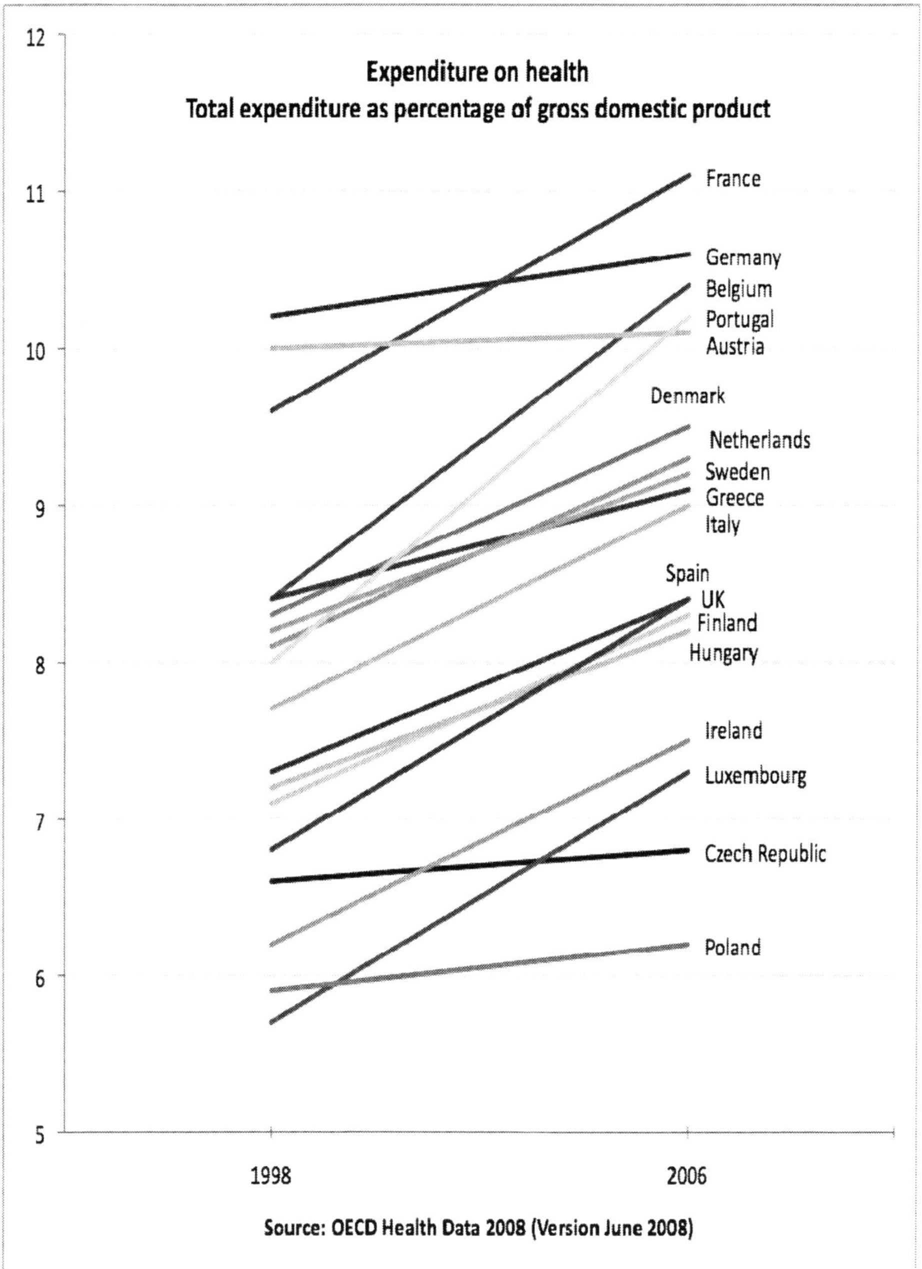

Figure 3: Total expenditure on health as a % of gross domestic product in EU countries[26]

26. http://ec.europa.eu/health/ph_information/dissemination/echi/echi_25_en.pdf.

Although the contribution from private financing is also increasing, the community covers the major part of health care costs.

Detailed information on national costs of undernutrition is rare. Nonetheless, the problem has become urgent. A survey in the UK of the number of visits or hospital admissions per person (> 65 years) per year shows that GP visits increased from 4.31 in non-undernourished people (low risk using MUST) to 7.10 in undernourished people. Likewise, hospital outpatient visits increased from 1.02 to 1.36 and hospital admissions from 0.28 to 0.50 with an increase in length of hospital stay of 30%.[xxvii]

Undernutrition-related disease is an economic burden in most countries, although limited data are available. Most of the data on the national cost of undernutrition are gathered in different countries in different care settings at different times using different criteria for undernutrition. An estimate for the UK shows that in 2003 public expenditure on disease-related undernutrition was €10.95 billion per year, or ≥ 10% of public expenditure on health. [xxviii] In Belgium the estimate is €400 million per year.[iii] In most cases, these costs are for the patients to pay. Since they are only in some cases partially reimbursed and often not at all, treatments are mostly cancelled or terminated early.

This confirms that undernutrition, although far from being recognised as an important health care problem, ranks in the same range of health care cost as obesity and overweight, conditions that are at the centre of all national health policies. Preventive medicine should therefore be one of the cornerstones of the actions undertaken to reduce health care costs (see Figure 4).[xxix]

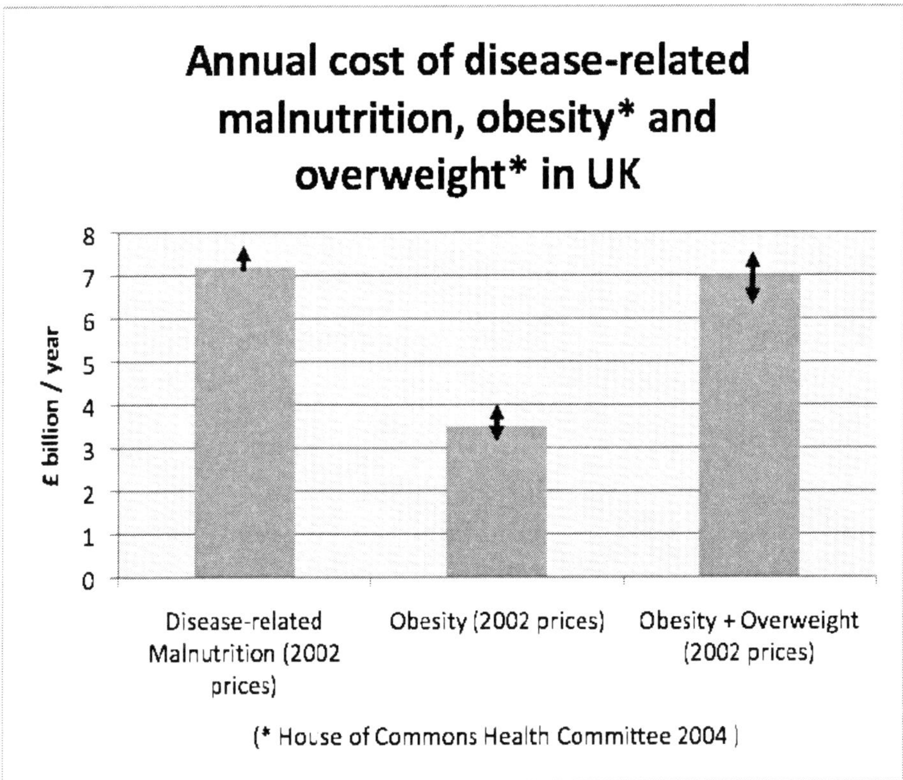

Figure 4: Annual cost of disease-related malnutrition, obesity and overweight in UK[27]

It is clear that most of the expenditure on disease-related malnutrition involves people over 65, who account for only about 15% of the general population. About half the cost of undernutrition occurs outside hospitals mainly for long-term residential care for older people.[xxvii]

Cost-effectiveness and cost-benefit assessment

To determine where and how to spend their money, public health services make a cost-effectiveness analysis, comparing the relative costs and outcomes of two or more courses of action. An example of this is cost-utility analysis, where the effects are measured in terms of years of full health lived. Low costs are always more easily accepted than high costs.

---

27. House of Commons Health Committee, "Obesity. Third report of session 2003-04. Volume 1", 27 May 2004, www.publications.parliament.uk/pa/cm200304/cmselect/cmhealth/23/23.pdf. Date of consultation: 27 October 2008.

However, the private coverage of costs is often ignored in these models, as well as the quality of life, the cost to caregivers and equity.

There is a clear need for a cost-effectiveness analysis, which should take into account social justice and an appropriate equity-efficiency trade-off.[xxviii]

A first way to reduce costs can be found in making hospital stays shorter. This can be done by assessing nutritional deficiencies at an early stage – and thus developing efficient screening methods in all health settings (see Chapter 7) and by addressing the problem adequately through the provision of nutritional support. Cost-effectiveness is not a simple task when it takes into account the various factors. Nonetheless, different attempts have been made, all suggesting that nutritional support is both cost-effective and cost-beneficial. However, these calculations should be extended and performed by experts in health economics. It is also important to take functional capability and an individual's satisfaction with their own life into account.

The choice of nutritional support determines treatment costs. In addition, the cost required to avoid complications and an extended length of stay should be balanced against the cost of providing aggressive artificial nutritional support unnecessarily.

The costs of the food service system can be divided into the costs of the initial design and construction of the food service premises, the distribution system, the serving premises and the day-to-day "running costs". The costs also vary according to the preparation system (new technologies, consultants, etc.). Specific European data for the total costs of food service are scarce, although it is known that the money spent on food is only a very small fraction of the total hospital budget.

As far as artificial feeding is concerned, substantial savings can be made through a better management of its practices. In general, it all comes down to using the most appropriate kind of support; for example, not using parenteral nutrition when enteral nutrition is more appropriate. In a number of countries the usefulness of protein-rich supplemental foods is recognised for therapeutic, but not yet for preventive, use. Reimbursement can help overcome the financial constraints older people often have.

Institution-related undernutrition and its costs could furthermore be reduced simply by a better overall food provision in hospitals and care homes.

Influence of the health cost finance structure

The structure of health care financing is an important factor in the adequate managing of nutritional support. In the hospital or nursing home, the costs of nutritional intervention with parenteral nutrition are often part of the medical care budget, while the costs for enteral nutrition (tube and sip) are part of the kitchen budget. It may not even be part of the normal financing for food and be charged separately to the patient. Parenteral nutrition (TPN) provided at home may be reimbursed to the patient or charged to the hospital budget where enteral products may not or only partially be reimbursed and have to be financed by the patients. The same holds true for the feeding and enteral supply equipment. Where home nutritional support by TPN is given, the hospital staff may provide dietetic and nursing advice whereas this is less likely for dietetic advice on enteral feeding, which may have to come from the individual. As the rate of complications, of compliance with the prescribed regimes, both in terms of frequency and quantity of feeding, and of hospital readmission is highly dependent on the care and knowledge of both the person and the caregiver, adequate information, individual coaching and technical and social support are needed.

Quality of life of the caregiver

When assessing costs of health care, another aspect that is almost consistently ignored is the quality of life and cost to the caregiver. In the UK, one in every eight people is a caregiver. This represents in the UK alone some 6 million people, mainly women, who are an invisible health care system on their own. It is estimated that 85 000 caregivers provide care for more than fifty hours per week and three out of five of all caregivers receive no regular visitor support services. Some 79% of caregivers say that the care they provide to the person they care for affects their health. Most of the complaints relate to backache (50%), stress/worry (91%) and depression (58%).

Specific recommendations with regard to the impact of undernutrition on health care costs:

- invest in policies that allow older people to stay at home; 95% of older people want to stay at home and, moreover, it represents a lower social cost for society;
- consider treatment of undernutrition either by parenteral or enteral nutrition as a medical act and therefore as part of the medical/pharmacy budget and not the kitchen budget;
- enable a smooth and accurate transition of people treated for undernutrition from hospital to other settings by lowering costs for the individual concerned (reimbursement of dietetic counselling and supplemental foods (parenteral, enteral, sip)).

5. Assessing and treating undernutrition in care homes and home care

Summary

- screening is the first step in assessing and treating undernutrition. The following tools are proposed: (1) Mini Nutritional Assessment (MNA) as the first screening choice; (2) the Malnutrition Universal Screening Tool (MUST) can be second; and (3) Subjective Global Assessment (SGA) is considered as the optimal tool for further nutritional assessment. The choice of the screening tool may depend on national practices and practical considerations of the setting;
- screening should be performed on admission to the nursing home and on a regular basis thereafter;
- nutritional support should be initiated by providing dietary advice and/or fortified foods, in collaboration with a dietician;
- in case of impossible or inadequate oral intake, artificial nutrition should be given, mainly by enteral nutrition. Ethical consideration is required for people with dementia.

Undernutrition is not the only factor responsible for all the physical and psychical changes seen in older people, but muscle depletion and undernutrition are undoubtedly a very important factor that can contribute to their development. Therefore, the treatment of older people should be efficient, without any delay due to dispensable diagnostic procedures. It should be kept in mind that each day spent in a hospital bed can significantly decrease the patient's chance of recovery. Proper nutrition should be started immediately, because body protein reserves are often relatively low and muscle tissue loss can play an important role in patient survival. Therefore, routine screening and nutritional assessment should be considered on a frequent basis, and food intake should be measured daily. Nutritional support should be provided without any delay if the standard intake is low. Physical rehabilitation (active or passive) should also be started as soon as possible, in order to ensure muscle activity.

Nutritional support should not be seen in isolation. When treating undernutrition, it is necessary to look beyond the nutritional status, and also address the underlying causes of undernutrition. Specific attention should be paid to mental diseases caused by undernutrition.

Nutritional risk screening and nutritional assessment

The first and main step to start addressing undernutrition in all health care settings is screening. It is well known that the number of people detected with, or at risk of, undernutrition increases markedly when screening procedures are implemented.[xxx]

The continuous progress of a nutritional care programme with nutritional risk screening may be able to improve the health outcomes of geriatric patients: a Belgian quality research programme has shown that hospital stays were significantly lower during the intervention period than during the observation period.[xxxi] The mean serum prealbumin concentration was also higher during this period. Other studies have shown that nutritional support reduces the risk of complications, shortens the length of stay and reduces mortality.

It is clear that nutritional screening is of major importance. Screening and nutritional assessment should therefore be part of routine practice. A comprehensive screening tool is clearly needed. The difficulty resides in finding the most appropriate screening method. This method must, however, be clinically relevant and cost effective to perform. The issue is that many studies do not take the severity and seriousness of the illness into account. It is therefore important to use proper measures, such as weight loss, BMI and (recent) food intake, as well as information regarding fluid balance, gastrointestinal symptoms, etc. In older people, age-related changes in body composition should not be neglected. Efficient screening for undernutrition should therefore consider factors such as the identification of the risk factors of undernutrition, an estimation of appetite and/or (recent) food intake, the measurement of body weight, the evaluation of weight loss and the calculation of parameters of body mass, such as BMI.

In Belgium, a group of scientific experts in undernutrition has stated that, in care homes and home care, Mini Nutritional Assessment (MNA)[xxxii, xxxiii] is the first screening choice. The Malnutrition Universal Screening Tool (MUST)[xxxiv] can be second, whilst Subjective Global Assessment (SGA)[xxxv] was considered as the optimal tool for further nutritional assessment (see appendix).

Screening the nutritional risk is the first step in the treatment process. The screening will be followed by a nutritional assessment. The goal is to identify people who have, or are at risk of developing, deficiencies of energy, protein or specific nutrients; to try to quantify these deficiencies and the risk of developing complications related to undernutrition and to monitor and adjust the adequacy of nutritional support. It should therefore be executed at an early stage and repeated regularly. Ideally, the screening method and its outcomes should be scientifically documented for predicting the clinical course of people fulfilling certain criteria. The method used should be easy to apply and intuitively understandable.

The most important weakness in the process of screening is appropriate weighing routines. Older people should be weighed in general practice during each consultation. In care homes, weighing should be performed on admission, then at least once weekly in hospitals, once every fifteen days for rehabilitative care, and once monthly during long-term care. The unavailability of measuring equipment, the lack of time and immobility of the person often makes routine weighing a real challenge. Furthermore, factors that may influence the interpretation of results, such as dehydration, oedema or fluid effusions, are not always sufficiently considered when interpreting the weight evolution. Special attention should also be given to measuring the height of elderly persons. Due to age, height may change significantly and may be difficult to measure.

Nutritional support, treatment, monitoring and follow-up

If a person is at risk or is suffering from undernutrition, a treatment plan should be developed, based on the person's nutritional status and spontaneous food energy and protein intake. It should also take into account the nature and severity of any underlying disease(s) and associated disabilities, as well as their probable outcomes (swallowing disorders, for example). The support must also integrate residents and close relatives' preferences as well as ethical considerations. It should be based on an accurate estimation of the energy and protein requirements, the immediate and long-term goals of the nutritional support, the routes appropriate for use of feeding, the anticipated duration of treatment and the discharge plan or home training. The residents and their relatives should be consulted in decisions regarding the goals of the treatment.

Apart from situations contraindicating oral feeding, nutritional support should, as a priority, be initiated by providing dietary advice and/or fortified foods, if possible in collaboration with a dietician.

Nutritional support should be initiated by providing dietary advice and other corrective measures. If possible, nutritional support should be similar to normal food intake. This means that more appropriate meal patterns and menus are necessary to meet the frequent small meal habits. It may also be necessary to modify the food texture according to the person's chewing and swallowing abilities, and to assist feeding when required. The pleasure of oral feeding can furthermore be helped by good oral health and by creating a better ambience during meals.

The simplest and safest way for nutritional support is eating more ordinary food, in some cases fortified by adding cream, milk, oil and similar ingredients, resulting in increased energy and protein intake (energy-dense menus). The use of snacks or supplemental foods between regular meals is important, especially in older people, because activities connected with food intake can positively stimulate the rehabilitation process. Portion sizes should be reduced and the energy and protein density of the food increased.

It may be necessary to provide specific training to cooks on how to prepare tasty meals with a high nutritional value. It is shown that especially proteins (given as protein supplements) may increase muscle proteosynthesis in undernourished older persons. Therefore protein-dense supplements might be preferred for this group of people. The latest Cochrane meta-analysis showed that oral supplements produce a small but consistent weight gain in older people.[xxxvi] There may also be a beneficial effect on mortality. However, it did not show evidence of improvements in clinical outcome, functional benefit or a reduction in length of hospital stay. Additional data from large-scale multi-centre trials would be required.

Oral supplements may be indicated in particular when dietary advice seems to be insufficient and enteral nutrition may be attempted if adequate oral nutrition support is impossible. In order to achieve optimal results, it is important that nutritional support continues after discharge from hospital.

It is often insufficiently acknowledged that the main source of nutrition and nutritional support comes from the normal meals that are served. These meals are often jeopardised by various diagnostic and treatment activities.[xxxvii] Particular attention should be paid to this because of the decline with age of the two components of taste, namely olfaction and the taste buds. This increase in taste thresholds suggests a need for richer tastes of food for older people. However, there are no satisfactory research data related to food palatability in older people and future research should be therefore devoted to this part of nutritional care in older people.

Isolated deficiencies of protein and micronutrients may also be observed even in older subjects apparently in good health. It is well known that older people are at risk of micronutrient deficiency (mainly group B vitamins, vitamin C, vitamin D, selenium, zinc and calcium, etc.).[xxxviii] Such deficiencies should also be addressed as appropriate.

Regular physical activity to prevent muscle wasting is as necessary as nutritional support. This can be done mainly by the fact that muscle activity is frequently low and immobilisation decreases the positive effect of nutritional support on the quality of life, concomitant disease and mortality.[xxxix]

French guidelines state that undernourished older subjects should achieve an energy intake of 30 to 40 Kcal/kg/day and a protein intake of 1.2 to 1.5 g/kg/day.[xl] Nutritional requirements, however, vary from individual to individual and must be adapted to comorbidities.

Several measures are recommended to increase food intake in older people in the French National Food and Health Plan (PNNS):[xli]

- increase eating frequency during the day by splitting up meals (with a minimum of three meals a day) and by proposing snacks between meals;
- do not allow the person to go without food for too long during the night (> twelve hours) by delaying dinner and advancing breakfast and/or by proposing a snack;
- provide mainly high-energy and/or high-protein foods;
- design menus to suit personal preferences and modify food texture according to chewing and swallowing ability;
- organise technical and/or human assistance for feeding according to a person's disabilities;
- provide meals in pleasant surroundings (dining room and companions).

In the case of underlying diseases and the presence of dementia, the nutritional requirements and concerns change as a disease progresses. While prior to the diagnosis, a normal, balanced diet may be indicated to maintain health, with the progression of the disease, wasting becomes more important and changing tastes, food habits and preferences may require appropriate adaptation of the nutritional support strategy.

The follow-up should be based on the periodic measurement of body weight and an estimation of food intake.

An example of a recommendation for a nutritional strategy is given below in Figure 5.[xviii]

Spontaneous dietary intake	Nutritional status: Normal	Nutritional status: Malnutrition	Nutritional status: Severe malnutrition
Normal	Monitoring	Dietary advice Fortified diet Reassessed at one month	Dietary advice Fortified diet and ONS Reassessed at fifteen days
Reduced but more than half of usual intake	Dietary advice Fortified diet Reassessed at one month	Dietary advice Fortified diet Reassessed at fifteen days and if failure: ONS	Dietary advice Fortified diet and ONS Reassessed at one week and if failure: EN
Very reduced and less than half of normal intake	Dietary advice Fortified diet Reassessed at one week and if failure: ONS	Dietary advice Fortified diet and ONS Reassessed at one week and if failure: EN	Dietary advice Fortified diet and EN from outset Reassessed at one week

Figure 5: Guideline on nutritional support in relation to food intake (ONS: oral nutritional supplements/EN: enteral nutrition)[28]

Nutritional support in dementia and the final stages of life

Nutritional support in dementia and the final stages of life presents an important ethical dilemma. The patient or resident, the caregiver and the health care professional may have different expectations and perceptions with regard to nutrition.[xlii]

In the moderate stage, memory loss can lead to missed meals, dehydration or, on the contrary, over-eating. Changes in food preferences may lead to undernutrition. For these reasons, it is important to be extremely vigilant. Caregivers may need guidance on how to ensure that the person with dementia has a healthy and balanced diet. But when dealing with nutrition, issues such as autonomy, choice and people's values should not be underestimated. In some care homes, meals are provided in the form of

---

28. Haute Authorité de Santé, "Clinical Practice Guidelines. Nutritional support strategy for protein-energy malnutrition in the elderly", April 2007, www.has-sante.fr/portail/upload/docs/application/pdf/malnutrition_elderly_guidelines.pdf, p. 8. Date of consultation: 27 October 2008.

buffets that give people with dementia the opportunity to retain their autonomy and exercise personal choice at mealtimes.

Good oral health through routine mouth care is important to maintain the pleasure of oral feeding. All symptoms that may reduce the desire to eat or the pleasure of eating, such as pain, nausea, glossitis and dryness of the mouth should be relieved.

In the advanced stage of dementia, difficulties to eat by natural means are not uncommon and some people simply stop eating. This might be due to badly fitting dentures but could reflect a deeper ethical issue, such as the expression of the person's will or his/her wish to die. This can be very difficult for caregivers to cope with. The medical team is also faced with the decision of whether to feed the person artificially and if so, by what method.

In the final stages of life, loss of weight as well as of muscle and muscle strength is common. People may also experience increasing difficulty in swallowing (known as dysphagia) as dementia worsens, resulting in a risk of aspiration (when food or liquid enters into the airway below the true vocal cords). This can increase the risk of aspiration pneumonia.

The question of how to feed the person and the role of artificial feeding is not an easy one. It is not always successful, it increases the risk of complications, and it is often considered with mixed emotions by caregivers. The emotional pressure on the medical team and the caregivers to take a decision on whether to initiate medically assisted feeding or rather to withhold food cannot be underestimated. Considerations such as "We can't let him/her die of hunger", "We can save him/her", "We've got to do something; otherwise it's the end" are counterbalanced by the observation that forced feeding is highly uncomfortable or goes against the will of the person.

There are definitely ethical dilemmas linked to the use of tube feeding and the withdrawal of food and liquid, for example debates on whether withholding food or resorting to tube feeding is beneficial or maleficent, at what point withholding food cannot be considered as the actual cause of death, prior wishes with regard to tube feeding, etc. Caregivers may be distressed if the person with terminal dementia can no longer take food and liquid and is not being tube fed. Clearly, there is a need for health care professionals to provide understandable information and to address these anxieties. The Alzheimer's Society is active in this field with several projects (for example, circle of care, self-help and discussions groups, Alzheimer's

Cafés, numerous publications and practical tips published on the website).[xliii]

Shapiro points to weaknesses in studies that showed that tube feeding did not prolong life in people with severe dementia. His own research supports other studies indicating that supportive care and tube feeding may extend life by months or even years.[xliv] Nevertheless, the Alzheimer's Society (UK), in its position paper on palliative care, states that the use of a tube for artificial hydration and feeding should not be considered best practice in the care of people in the advanced stage of dementia.[xliii]

By providing practical assistance in eating and food choice, one should in principle be able to delay the introduction of artificial feeding, but of course it takes a great amount of time and a lot of patience to adapt to the person's speed and eating habits. Education and encouragement of caregivers is therefore a very important aspect to improve care and nutritional support. Summersall recommends that health care professionals receive training in how to perform swallowing assessments and in adopting appropriate tailored interventions.[xlv] Management strategies include, for example, advice to nursing staff and caregivers on swallowing, modifying the diet, using food in purée form and thick liquids, correct positioning and feeding strategies. Patience, gentle encouragement, knowing the person's eating habits, adapting to his/her speed and social interaction are also important and need time. According to the National Council for Palliative Care (NCPC), good food given by skilled caregivers to people with dementia often obviates the need for medical dietary support.[xlvi] Unfortunately, professional caregivers do not always have the necessary time to provide this kind of quality care.

The primary objectives of nutritional support during the last weeks of life of an older person should be pleasure and comfort. Having recourse to the parenteral or enteral routes is not recommended, especially as intubation may be a source of discomfort. This decision must be explained to the nursing team and the person's close relatives.

Recommendations:

- have multi-stakeholder discussions on the best ways of artificial feeding in ill older people;
- organise education of the caregivers on the specific skills needed.

The hospital-care home-home care continuum

Undernutrition is often present but not recognised before hospital admission. During hospitalisation, undernutrition is known to aggravate because of chronically insufficient food intake and inefficient nutritional support. People themselves often have a limited knowledge of the adverse effects of undernutrition and are not provided with the necessary contact information to help them cope with their nutritional difficulties. This results in a further aggravation of their situation, and dramatically increases the risk of re-hospitalisation. The only way to break this futile cycle is by a "continuum of care" at home and in the hospital, which can only be achieved by an overall increase in the awareness of undernutrition;[iv] the person and his/her relatives should also be better informed by an information campaign on the risks related to undernutrition. This information should be included in the training of all health care professionals.

As described above, one can only obtain optimal results when nutritional support is continued after discharge from hospital. Close co-operation between home care personnel, general practitioners, food services, etc., is therefore mandatory. The nutritional status and information on nutritional support should be included in a person's records. Nutritional support should, furthermore, also be extended to pre-hospitalisation periods. Undernutrition should be an important element for local general practitioners and home care organisations to screen for.

Specific recommendations with regard to the assessment and treatment of undernutrition in care homes and home care:

- put at the disposal of care homes simple and efficient tools to detect undernutrition. Such tools should be evidence-based and validated in these settings. They ought to be simple, easy to use and feasible and they should take into account the relevant characteristics of the individual. They also should enable easy identification of people at risk or suffering from undernutrition;
- establish methods of reference, based upon the criteria listed above (cf. recommended methods for screening and nutritional assessment of the Belgian Food and Health Plan);
- nutritional screening should be performed on all residents in a continuous manner;

- establish a structured and multidisciplinary approach towards systematic and individual nutritional assessment, treatment and follow-up of people that have been identified as being at risk or suffering from undernutrition;
- such nutritional assessment should include specialised personnel (dietician), the identification of an individual's nutritional needs, the correction of physical, psychological and social factors impeding adequate food intake, and the systematic monitoring of food intake, body weight and other relevant parameters;
- in smaller institutions where it may be too expensive to employ a dietician on a full-time basis, a mobile nutrition support team, working in one or several institutions, could help to organise nutritional support and ensure nutrition according to evidence-based criteria;
- provide high quality meals (taste and nutritional value), in dialogue with the council of residents for the composition of the menus;
- select food services delivering high quality meals to the homes of older people;
- the threshold for nutritional interventions with specialised supplemental foods (foods for special medical purposes) should be lowered by reimbursing such foods where indicated in care homes and home care;
- nutritional support, started in hospital, should continue in care homes and home care and for a sufficiently long period;
- health care workers should be vigilant for socioeconomic variables interfering with appropriate nutritional support, for example, social isolation, apathy, mental conditions, motor and dental problems, and financial constraints. Therefore, screening should be repeated at regular intervals in care homes as well as in home care by medical/paramedical staff;
- nutritional support should be monitored and efficiently tailored in order to achieve clear goals;
- medical records and medical discharge letters should contain information on an individual's nutritional status and physical and mental condition in relation to food intake. Such information should accompany the person in a systematic way between the different settings and be accessible by all health care workers involved;

- a person's weight and height as well as nutritional interventions should be part of their medical file in all settings (hospitals, care homes and home care);
- a co-ordinated multidisciplinary structure involving all stakeholders is needed to pilot these nutritional objectives in home care settings.

6. Strategies to tackle undernutrition in hospitals

Although the situation in hospitals is not the subject of this report, as it was addressed by the Council of Europe in its report on food and nutritional care in hospitals in 2002, it is nevertheless important to recall the major barriers to proper nutritional care that were identified in the hospital setting.[i] In particular, undernutrition often exists prior to admission and can be provoked or aggravated through hospitalisation. Family doctors must therefore attach great importance to a person's dietary habits, and their diet must be assessed at admission, and systematically screened during their stay at hospital.

The Council of Europe report identified five factors that seem to be the major barriers to proper nutritional care in hospitals in Europe.[xlvii]

The first is the lack of clearly defined responsibilities in the planning and management of nutritional care. These responsibilities should be clearly defined and assigned by setting standards for practice in view of assessing and monitoring the nutritional risk and status of the patient. Furthermore, responsibility regarding the nutritional care and support of patients should not be limited to the hospital stay (continuum of care).

A second factor is the lack of sufficient education on nutrition and its role among all staff groups, which makes it hard to recognise or treat disease-related undernutrition.[xlviii] There seems to be a gap between what is being taught and the results of nutritional research. This makes it difficult to provide optimal nutritional support according to the principles of best-documented practice, although the vast majority of those concerned are convinced that clinical nutrition should be a recognised specialism. A general improvement in education is undoubtedly required, specifically a continuing educational programme on general nutrition and techniques of nutritional support and monitoring. This should focus on the nutritional training of non-clinical staff, as well as on the definitions of their area of responsibility. A "European advanced course in clinical research" has already been launched by ESPEN (the European Society for Clinical Nutrition and Metabolism), as well as a programme for nutritional education in medical schools by the Federation of European Nutrition Societies (FENS). Nurses seem to have the greatest lack of knowledge, and have admitted that they find it difficult to identify patients at risk, set up nutrition plans and monitor their effects. Non-clinical staff, often helping nurses on the wards, also have a great lack of nutritional knowledge, although they have the closest contact with the patient when it comes to food intake. Clinical and general dieticians seem to receive the most up-to-date training. Their role, however, varies widely throughout Europe. Finally, the kitchen staff should also receive proper training with regard to energy-dense meals for undernourished patients, in order to make these meals available in every hospital.

Furthermore, there seems to be a lack of influence from patients, which can be traced back to poor knowledge of the food issue. Patients should have the possibility of individualising their meals and ordering (extra) food. They should also be involved in the planning of their meals and have the possibility to give feedback to develop appropriate, target-specific menus. Studies have already shown that food consumption can be improved without a change of menu, if the patients are involved in planning their meals, have some control over the selection of food and feel responsible for following the advice given. Information campaigns on the importance of good nutrition for successful treatment prior to admission and after discharge should also be considered and set up.

Lack of co-ordination between different staff groups is another barrier. These groups (managers, physicians, dieticians, nurses, etc.) should all work together in order to achieve optimal patient care from the nutritional point of view. This co-operation should be considered as a priority and should be optimised by the hospital management. The latter should also look into organised contacts between the hospital and the first-line health care workers. A so-called “nutritional support team” can establish co-operation between the different caregiver groups. Numerous studies have already proven their benefits when it comes to securing the nutrient requirements of the patients and saving money. It could co-ordinate the food service system and nutritional support, set standards for nutritional risk screening, develop protocols for action to be undertaken, implement an audit process, etc. Communication between the various groups could be co-ordinated by a contact person, who could also co-ordinate communication between the hospital and the primary health care sector, which ensures follow-up on the patient’s condition.

A final common barrier is the lack of involvement of hospital management. The revision of meals should be considered as an important part in the treatment process, and the hospital management should therefore take responsibility for delivering an appropriate food service and nutritional care to their patients, and give priority to food policy and the management of food services. When meals are not produced in-house, hospitals should develop standards and guidelines for outsourcing food service. Management should therefore prioritise the creation of an organisational framework in which food service and nutritional issues can be discussed, next to setting up a quality management system to ensure the quality of the food that is produced and presented. When assessing the costs of the food service, they should take into account the costs of complications and prolonged hospital stays due to undernutrition.

More specifically, the Belgian National Food and Health Plan has already proposed installing a nutrition manager and a nutrition committee in each hospital, as well as setting up the National Group of Experts on Undernutrition.

The nutrition manager should be a specialist doctor with expertise in nutrition. He/she should install a nutrition committee, which can assist the nutrition manager in – among other things – defining a global policy on nutrition, setting up systematic screening and assessment tools and scientific intervention procedures and rigorous monitoring of the institutional food services. The committee should also guarantee professional development on nutrition and determine the necessary resources.

The National Group of Experts on Undernutrition was set up at federal level to establish scientific lines of conduct on standardised methodologies for screening and monitoring, draft advice related to the necessary measures and means for applying the proposed lines of conduct, and give advice on the form, measures and budgets necessary for sharing the costs of nutritional intervention.

Specific recommendations in relation to the hospital setting have been identified and formulated in the 2002 report.[i]

7. Strategies to tackle undernutrition in care homes and home care

Summary

- a multidisciplinary approach is important to successfully tackle undernutrition on multiple levels: the undernourished person, the health care workers (medical and non-medical), the caregivers, the public, policy makers and society stakeholders;
- awareness for the person, health care professionals and caregivers is important; this can be secured by information and appropriate training;
- care home management and kitchen staff activities can be modified in order to promote nutrition;
- policy makers should create legal frameworks to confront undernutrition as a public health concern.

Raising awareness

Raising awareness and increasing recognition of undernutrition requires a multifactorial approach and should focus on two levels: the health care workers, including non-medical staff involved with food and patient care, and the public (see Figure 6).[xxvi] To tackle the issue of undernutrition, it is important that every link in the patient care chain is aware of the problem and acknowledges its role in the multidisciplinary approach.

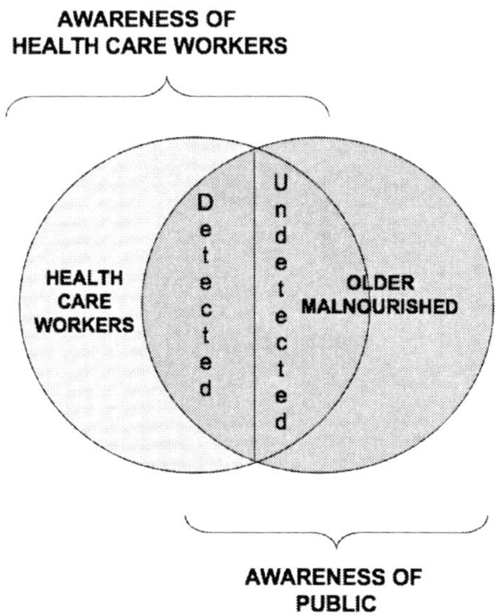

Figure 6: Awareness – A shared responsibility[29]

Nutritional information to health care professionals and caregivers is an essential measure, not only to raise awareness but also to share science-based practices. Such information may take the form of guidelines, quality improvement programmes, charters or recommendations specifying responsibilities, required structures, screening and nutritional assessment routines, training courses, etc.

A second element is of course that despite the existence of guidelines and recommendations, the target audience must be:

- aware of the existence of these materials;
- read and process it; and
- implement it.

Experience shows that lack of instruments, time and administrative support are the main reasons why such guidelines are often not or only partially implemented, unless such measures are part of the legislative provisions in order to meet criteria for financing (see Figure 7).[xlix]

29. Elia, M., "Malnutrition in older people", www.fhf.org.uk/meetings/2006-03-21_presentation_elia.pdf, p. 2. Date of consultation: November 2008.

	1997	2004
Lack of knowledge	54% (418)	48% (636)
Lack of interest	50% (389)	47% (632)
Lack of defined responsibility	45% (348)	45% (601)
Lack of documentation (of effect)	23% (183)	25% (329)
Time consuming	17% (129)	36% (487)
Difficult to identify relevant patients	31% (241)	13% (172)
Too expensive	8% (60)	6% (81)
Too many complications (to nutrition therapy)	4% (29)	7% (94)
Technically difficult	4% (29)	4% (59)
Other	14% (113)	14% (185)
Total*	249% (780)	245% (1340)

*More than one answer was permitted

Figure 7: Reasons why nutrition therapy is often not or only partially implemented[30]

This means that even the most basic principles for preventing undernutrition are not implemented. Some examples are :

– despite the fact that sufficient food intake is a basic requirement of proper nutrition, experience from the Nutrition Day project shows that on the day of the survey, 50% of people were not eating an adequate quantity of food (see Figure 8).[I]

30. Lindorff-Larsen, K. et al., "Management and perception of hospital undernutrition – A positive change among Danish doctors and nurses", *Clinical Nutrition*, 26 (3), 2007, pp. 371-378.

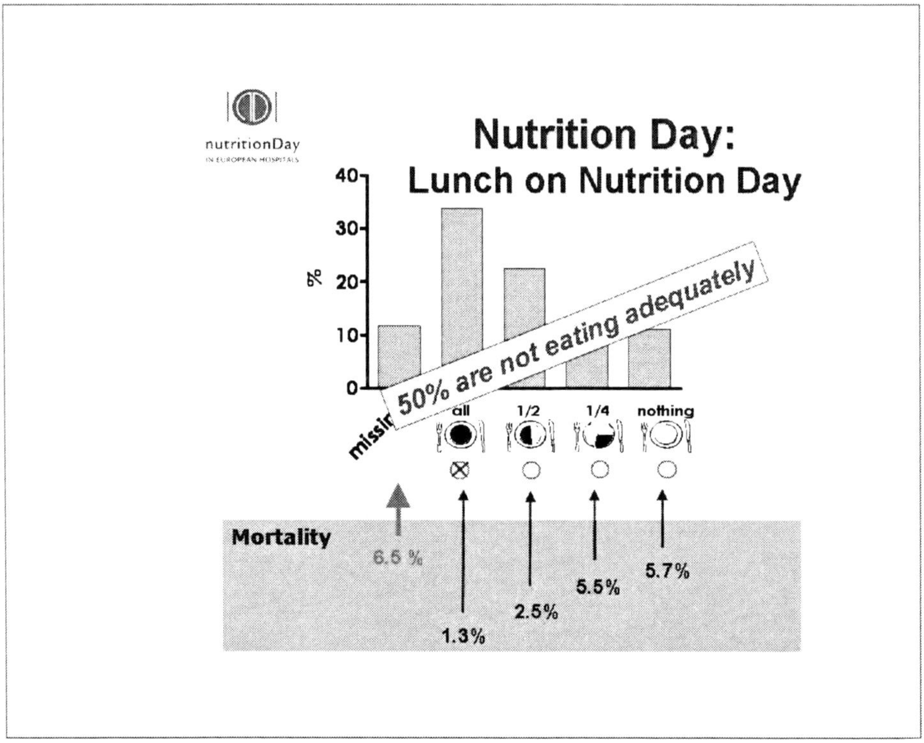

Figure 8: Meal consumption linked to mortality[31]

– despite the obvious observation that people with low body weight are more prone to being undernourished, the Nutrition Day shows that in the care home setting, 60% of residents with a BMI < 20 kg/m² were not recognised as undernourished (see Figure 9).[li]

31. Schindler, K., presentation at the Forum on Undernutrition in Care Homes and Home Care, November 2007, www.nutritionday.org.

60% of nursing home residents with a BMI < 20 kg/m² were not recognised as malnourished

	Malnutrition			
	Yes	Risk	No	Total
BMI < 20 kg/m²	131	96	61	**288**
BMI 20-22 kg/m²	24	72	140	**236**
BMI > 22 kg/m²	20	75	1094	**1189**
Total	**175**	**243**	**1295**	**1713**

Figure 9: Recognition of malnutrition in relation to BMI[32]

- experience from Germany illustrates that whereas it is well known that 25% of all admissions to hospital are undernourished patients and that this increases with age, information on nutritional status is included in the patient chart in only 30% of patients and nutritional therapy is only initiated in 10-30% of undernourished people;[lii]
- while it is well known that people move between hospital, care homes and home care, and that information on nutritional status and nutritional support that is initiated in one of the settings needs to be passed on to the next setting, a report from German insurance companies shows that data on nutritional status are missing in the majority of cases and that while the indication of tube feeding was correct in more than 90% of cases, the prescribed amount is too low and therapy control was inadequate;
- although there is much evidence to support a strong correlation between nutritional status and clinical outcome, it is apparent that scientific specialists, insurance companies, health care facilities and general practitioners just ignore these data. But things can improve as research from Denmark shows. A marked improvement in the situation was seen between 1997 and 2004 after guidelines had been

32. www.nutritionday.org/uploads/media/Valentini_Ernaehrung2007_01.pdf, p. 6. Date of consultation: 27 October 2008.

issued, pocket booklets distributed, study results reported and quality improvement programmes implemented.[xlvi]

It goes without saying that the success of implementing guidelines will also depend on factors relating to the perception of the undernourished person, which can be influenced by age, gender, race, religious conviction, socioeconomic status, insurance status, comorbidities, preferences, etc.

Finally, a lack of expertise, commitment and/or resources of the health care system or the health care system as a whole will also greatly determine the efficiency of implementing guidelines and recommendations. Clearly, guidelines and recommendations are required but without supportive measures they will only have limited effects, especially in care homes and home care.

Specific recommendations with regard to raising awareness:

- structural provisions in the health care system are required, with statutory measures tailored specifically to care homes and home care, supporting nutrition teams, imposing systematic screening, professional training and certification, etc.;
- financing modalities of care for individual undernourished people should be in relation to their screening in order to provide an incentive for care homes to perform systematic screening;
- greater financing for taking on board nutritional support of undernourished people and reimbursement of supplemental foods should be provided.

The roles and responsibilities of health care workers

The general practitioner – Family doctor

According to a study carried out by the British Association of Parenteral and Enteral Nutrition (BAPEN), a large number of general practitioners consider the measurement of body weight as unimportant. This study concluded that a solution might be found in specific training on nutrition with a focus on undernutrition. The Federation of European Nutrition Societies (FENS) initiated the development of such training for every medical student, either to be obtained during university training or during a postgraduate education programme.

The general practitioner is a key person with regard to providing information to their patients in care homes or at home, before admission to hospital and after their discharge. He/she is also the key person who should at all times be aware of the nutritional status of his/her patients. He/she should be able to describe basic aspects of food and nutrition, to describe the relationship between nutrition and health, to identify people at risk of developing nutrition-related diseases, to detect undernutrition through knowledge of the risk factors and diagnosis of the symptoms, and to prescribe appropriate nutritional support strategies.

Today, various associations and organisations provide this kind of training for general practitioners, so that they are capable of detecting undernutrition.

Specific recommendations in relation to fields of action and responsibility of the family doctor:

- implement continuing education programmes for general practitioners to make them aware of the continuous attention he/she should have for patients' nutritional status, even when the patient is seeking assistance for a non-related illness;
- include nutritional support in under- and postgraduate education of general practitioners;
- support initiatives to raise family doctors' awareness of undernutrition.

Care home and home care nursing staff

As in hospitals, the problem of undernutrition is not sufficiently known by nursing staff in care homes and home care. This observation is a direct consequence of the general lack of knowledge regarding nutrition and undernutrition per se. It can be attributed to the inadequacy of courses in this domain for the medical professions.

Basic courses in nutrition often do not exist in the regular retraining courses of GPs, specialists and nurses. Cross-disciplinary co-operation should be at the heart of training so that doctors and nursing staff can take appropriate measures and call upon specialist help (dieticians) more quickly.[liii]

Specific recommendations in relation fields of action and responsibility of nursing staff in the care home and home care environment:

- implement continuing education programmes on general nutrition and undernutrition and techniques of nutritional support for all staff involved in the feeding of patients, care home residents and old people at home;
- include nutritional support in under- and postgraduate courses for physicians, pharmacists and nurses, and other health care professionals involved in nutritional care;
- recognise the need for specific training in (clinical) nutrition, such as separate courses, chairs, postgraduate training, etc., and implement it in all medical schools;
- increase the nutritional training of non-clinical staff, as diagnosing signs of dysphagia, help with eating and monitoring of intake, weight and other parameters are essential in effective nutritional support.

The dietician

The dietician is at the centre of specialised nutritional care. His/her role and expertise are essential in the treatment of people at risk of or suffering from undernourishment.

Dieticians must provide effective, evidence-based nutritional assessment, dietary advice and support to patients, their caregivers and all staff involved in patient care.

Dieticians should provide nutritional training to nurses, doctors, health professionals and patients, not only in the context of undernutrition, but on all aspects of nutrition.

Although dieticians should have the most up-to-date knowledge on undernutrition, their educational level and responsibility are fairly low in practice. Moreover, it is clear that their role in nutritional management varies dramatically from country to country in Europe.

To regain the central place the dietician deserves, professional organisations of dieticians should address the quality of nutritional care and the role of the dietician at the European level. Minimal standards for education should be established. Standardisation of dieticians' levels of competence in the community setting is required, in order for the value of their profession in the management of undernutrition to be acknowledged.

Specific recommendations in this respect have been established by ESPEN, focusing on the hospital setting, with the overall intention of identifying minimum educational standards for the whole of Europe.[liv] ESPEN's recommendations include: (1) an agreement on the key functions of the clinical dietician working in nutritional support; (2) an identified programme of postgraduate study for clinical dieticians leading to specialisation in nutritional support; (3) a plan to develop and apply an accredited and integrated European standard in nutritional support. Such efforts should also be made in order to create a "community dietician".

Specific recommendation as regards the fields of action and responsibility of dieticians in the care home and home care environment:

- establish standards for the education and training of dieticians and improve the current level of education. Recognise the role of the dietician as the central person in nutritional support and teach responsibilities and skills, adapted to these needs;
- assign defined responsibilities and tasks to the dietician in the care home environment. Such responsibilities will include:
  - assuring that meals are nutritious and diversified and that good quality snacks and supplemental foods are available;
  - analysing menus, participating in the elaboration of recipes, and proposing alternatives in co-ordination with the cook and the appropriate financial manager;
  - assuring that the choice of meals gets larger, and organising this expansion of choice with the cook (planning, anticipation);
  - assuring the purchase of appropriate food in collaboration with the cook and the relevant financial manager;
  - controlling and adapting food portions so that each older person receives an adequate portion;
  - participating in a "council of residents" where residents can exchange views and opinions with the care home management regarding their care and other aspects of their stay;

- participating, in collaboration with the management and the cook, in an assessment of the residents' levels of satisfaction (on the basis of the advice of the council of residents);
- taking part in an assessment of correction measures in the field of food safety, together with kitchen staff, nurses and external organisations (food control agencies);
- taking part in a multidisciplinary approach to the nutritional follow-up of all residents; install, participate in and assess the screening of undernutrition;
- meeting frequently with the physician and the care home nurse to review the diets of undernourished residents;
- elaborating, in collaboration with the physician, the appropriate nutritional therapies, adapted to different situations and pathologies;
- participating in meal taking and, if necessary, helping the residents; assuring regular contact with each resident so that the nutritional response is personalised;
- proposing to management, staff members and residents all measures that are likely to establish a nutrition charter in the care home;
- facilitating, organising and assuring, in collaboration with the physician, the circulation of the nutritional records of each resident among the various parties involved in the care home, and in primary care;
- making sure that awareness-raising measures are put in place, and proposing training for the staff members concerned;
- participating in the decision-making process with regard to the organisation and environment of meal taking;
- making sure, together with management, that there is sufficient staff on duty during meal taking;
- taking part in the recruitment of staff concerned with nutrition and feeding;

- the dietician should be dedicated to playing his/her role as the central person in the nutritional care of people and sufficient time should be assigned to this task in order for it to be effective.

The roles and responsibilities of health care facilities

Care homes

An adequate nutritional state is essential for maintaining good health. Although in most cases food is presented in sufficient quantity and quality, care homes have a high percentage of residents in a state, or at risk, of undernutrition (40-80%).

The main cause is the lack of statutory provisions regarding the quality and quantity of meals, monitoring nutritional state, and the lack of structural mechanisms for managing a food policy and staff qualifications.

The second cause is – as is the case for hospitals – the lack of training of the staff, resulting in an ignorance of the nutritional needs of older people.

Further aspects include lack of time to invest in helping residents, inappropriate organisation and atmosphere during meal times, absence of protocols for nutritional monitoring and support, etc.

Furthermore, ageing itself interferes with identification of risk and nutritional management of undernourished people. The habitual signs of ageing and pathologies of older people mask the symptoms of undernutrition, making identification of people at risk difficult. Mental and physical dependency, diseases and medical problems and bad dentition and spoiled gums may seriously impair nutritional support.[lv]

In relation to these issues, the Belgian National Food and Health Plan has proposed to draw up a "nutrition quality charter", drafting criteria for audit accreditation, which is to be included in local, regional and federal legislation. These accreditation criteria should cover a written nutrition policy, documented and applied procedures or protocols for early detection, through screening and monitoring of the undernourished older person (regular weight and oral hygiene checks), the appointment of a qualified "quality and nutrition manager", a "food and nutrition liaison committee" (drafting of procedures and protocols, working documents, audits, etc.), a pleasant environment and favourable psychological ambience, and the provision of a healthy and balanced diet, which includes the availability of individual and suitable food servings, all checked by the quality and nutrition manager. Furthermore, the residents' individual (nutritional) needs should be integrated and appropriate training of staff should be guaranteed.

An example of the usefulness and effectiveness of simple and practical interventions can be found in the Zorg voor Beter improvement project "Eating and Drinking", conducted in the Netherlands in 2006-07.[lvi] The goal of this project is to lower the incidence of undernutrition by raising awareness about the importance of eating and drinking, the need for adequate food intake, as well as the need to create a pleasant environment during eating. It is based upon two interventions aimed at facilitating appetite/improving mealtime atmosphere and screening for undernutrition. Raising awareness is achieved by teaching the staff how to improve appetite and to optimise atmosphere during meal times. Changes in mealtime atmosphere include:

- respecting the appropriate times and duration of meals;
- providing a normal and familiar table setting (tablecloth, real glasses, normal plates (no plates divided into three sections), napkins, full cutlery, subtle flower arrangements, etc.);
- creating social and balanced dining groups that are able to choose what to eat at the table, starting and ending together and with the staff sitting at the table and stimulating conversations;
- not interrupting meals: namely, no administration of medication during eating, staff changeover, disturbances by doors opening and closing, people passing by, activities unrelated to the meal (for example, cleaning, doctors, visits).

Experience after one year shows an increased awareness of undernutrition and the importance of meals. This is exemplified by a reduction in the "island culture" (where care and kitchen staff operate separately, with no common purpose to improve quality). It also led to an increase in the number of wards with undernutrition protocols. Results from 2 300 residents showed (LPZ 2007 versus 2006) optimised mealtime ambience in 90% of the wards, increased screening for undernutrition in 71% of cases (= an increase of 3½ times more in one year) and a 50% reduction in serious loss of weight (> 3 kg in one month, > 6 kg in six months) in only 3.5% of wards. The number of wards where no measures were taken for residents who were undernourished decreased by 50% to 14%. The project resulted in a significant decrease in undernutrition (see Figure 10).

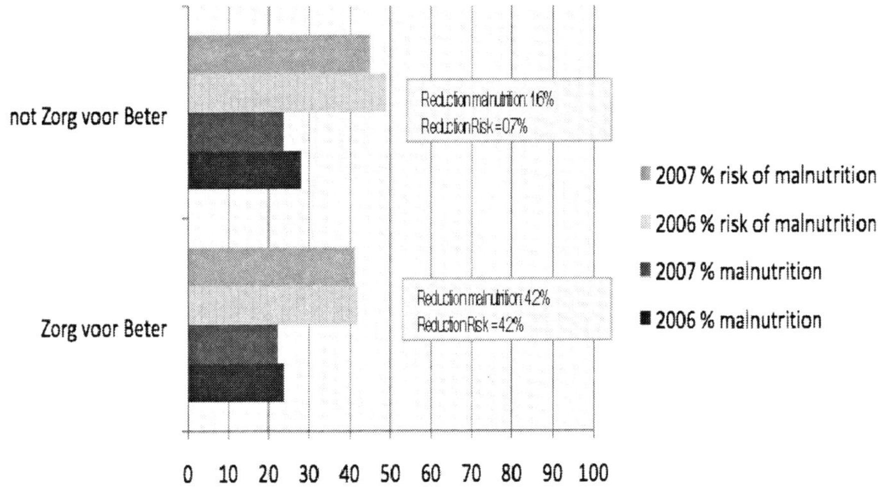

Figure 10: LPZ project: reduction of malnutrition between 2006 and 2007[33]

Specific recommendations with regard to strategies aimed at tackling undernutrition in care homes:

- the management of care homes should acknowledge their responsibility in relation to screening, nutritional assessment and nutritional care of residents;
- the management of care homes should acknowledge the importance of adequate food provisions, both in relation to quantity and quality, and provide for a pleasant eating environment and sufficient staff to help the residents who have problems during meals;
- care home management, physicians, pharmacists, nurses, dieticians and food service staff should work together in providing nutritional care and acknowledge food service as an important part of treatment and care of residents;
- there should be certification of care homes with good nutritional practice. Voluntary (cf. nutrition quality charter) and legal requirements relating to screening, nutritional support and quality of foods and services should be adhered to;
- a sufficient number of people involved in nutritional support, who are (partially) paid by the local authorities, should be available;

33. www.lpz-um.nl.

- the responsibility of different staff categories with respect to nutritional care and support and food service should be clearly assigned;
- in case of outsourcing of food services, guidelines and standards for food quality should be developed. Such contracts should be sufficiently detailed and cover special diets and personal preferences. Control should be in place to monitor the standards agreed;
- dieticians should be involved in all nutrition-related problems as the central person.

Standards for nutritional care and support in relation to costs, contract specifications, nutritional risk screening and audits should be established, for example, in the form of a nutritional charter that should contain the following requirements:

- put in place screening procedures as well as follow-up of nutritional support:
  - in the care homes, screening and follow-up of undernutrition must be taken into account in the global evaluation of health and its corrective measures. This should include regular weighing and oral hygiene checks at least once a month;
  - this involves the deployment of competent staff in sufficient numbers;
- require the presence of a "quality and nutrition manager", preferably with a bachelor's degree in nutrition and dietetics in every institution (full-time equivalent in relation to the number of residents). He/she:
  - looks after the quality of food and meals and is in charge of compliance with food hygiene standards;
  - takes part in the planning of menus and meals and participates in the purchasing of food and food supplements;
  - is in charge of the individual nutritional follow-up of every resident in dialogue with the attending physician or the co-ordinating doctor and nurses;
- elaboration of a "food and nutrition liaison committee", consisting of the professionals involved in food (cook, dietician, nurses, doctor, speech therapist, physiotherapist, occupational therapist). This committee:

- guarantees the flow of information concerning the nutritional condition and follow-up of older people between the (internal and external) people involved;
- puts in place protocols for the screening of undernutrition and the follow-up of undernourished older people;
- works out adequate food therapies, adapted to the various situations and pathologies;
- puts in place awareness-raising measures on undernutrition amongst all staff and the corresponding continuing education;

- create a pleasant environment and atmosphere during meals, including the possibility for residents to choose their dining environment and to sit at a table when eating their main meals. This implies:
  - sufficient staff are on duty during meals;
  - the presence of adequate equipment to help older people eat and drink; involve relatives and nursing staff to help the person eat;
- monitor satisfaction. Give older people the possibility of giving their opinion about the quality of meals and menus and take it into consideration;
- guarantee access to a healthy and balanced diet and inform residents and relatives, by means of leaflets, etc., of the nutritional care in the institution and the available dishes and foods:
  - offer menus and meals (according to nutritional recommendations) made and validated by a dietician;
  - offer sufficient choice. Provide a choice of foods in accordance with the residents' religious, ethnic and cultural backgrounds. Respect the food habits and preferences of older people. Offer individual servings adapted to the tastes and preferences of older people in order to offer them a tailor-made adequate meal. Provide the possibility to order snacks or supplemental foods at any time during the day. Provide for flexible and individualised meals. The standards for food service systems should be based on the needs of the resident rather than on the needs of the institution. Have a variety of snacks and nourishing drinks available and easily accessible between meals, to be offered whenever appropriate. Provide for a range of meals enriched in energy and protein;

- only prescribe diets with scientifically documented effects, keeping in mind the risk of undernutrition, which has to be closely monitored, and avoid fasting;
- encourage systematic feedback from the residents to the kitchen and ward staff in relation to the likes and dislikes of the food served;
- consider whether some people might benefit from vitamin/mineral supplementation, sip feeding or specific foods for special medical purposes and lower the financial threshold for reimbursement;

– elaborate standards for qualification and training of staff:

- provide appropriate training for non-medical staff on how to monitor food intake and how to provide for a user-friendly system for systematic recording of the quantity of food eaten at tray collection;
- provide specific qualifications for the profession of collective caterer and cook in a care home;
- establish a training programme that is specific to the old people sector and continuing education for all staff working in care homes, in particular on the issue of undernutrition amongst older people;
- organise a better flow of information among hospitals, care homes and home care, thereby ensuring improved nutritional follow-up thanks to "medical and nutritional records" or centralised electronic medical and nutritional patient records for all older people.

Food provision

An important observation is that many old people, not only those living in nursing homes, but also some living in private homes, do not eat enough to cover their needs. A French study, assessing food intake in several nursing homes in Auvergne, showed that 30-40% of residents, average age 87, eat less than 1 500 kcal/day and less than 30% achieve the French RDAs. At home, 11% eat less than 1 300 kcal/day and only 50% achieve the RDAs, even though they are younger, on average 79, and less dependent (see Figure 11).[xx]

		Percentage of old people from 12 Auvergne nursing homes (age 87.6 ± 4.7, male 25%, female 75%)	Percentage of self-sufficient elderly living at home (taken from a group of 987) (age 79 ± 5.2, male 35%, female 65%)
Calorie intake	< 1 300 kcal/day	Between 12% and 26%	11%
	1 300-2 000 kcal/day	Between 52% and 65%	37%
	> 2 000 kcal/day	Between 8% and 36%	52%

Figure 11: Intake of nutrients in French nursing homes and among old people living at home[34]

Reasons for insufficient intake have been widely studied in recent years. Ageing per se is linked to appetite modifications, including the inability of older people to appropriately react to intake stress, changes in taste and smell capacities, dental problems, etc. The presence of diseases in many of them also pushes them towards lower food consumption. In addition, physical disabilities, frequent at this age, are an additional handicap for food intake through the frequent inability to shop or to cook, the difficulty to cut meat or to chew hard dishes.

However, another factor is also the fact that prepared meals, particularly in homes, are not always appropriate for the capabilities or preferences of older people, generally because cooks have never been trained to take into account the needs and wishes of older people.

Several examples show that it is possible to increase food intake by simple measures and dedicated multidisciplinary programmes. In Denmark, an eleven-week intervention trial with several chocolate-based foods (compliance) and physical activity training significantly improved energy and protein intake and resulted in better weight parameters and nutritional status.[lvii] The physical activity programme resulted in significantly better scores in various physical tests.

In France, a special training programme was developed for cooks and caterers. They learn to make up a dish plan to achieve day-to-day adapted

34. Lesourd, B. et al., "Comment favoriser la prise alimentaire des sujets âgés?", *Nutr Clin Metabl*, 15, 2001, pp. 177-188.

food equilibrium for old people. They also learn how to prepare enriched food of better nutritional content compared to what is on the market, and also the quantity that needs to be served. The training emphasises in particular the preparation of tasty food, adapted to the taste of older people, in order to increase food intake.[xx]

Before training, the mixed dishes routinely prepared by cooks in homes, or served by an external organisation, comprise 230-250 kcal and 9-16 g of protein for a 200 g meat-vegetable mixed dish.

After training, preparations of a similar size dish (200 g) contain twice as many calories (nearly 500 kcal). In some homes, such preparations also contain more protein (+ 30 g), more calcium (+ 290 mg) and more fibre (+ 3 g). In addition, they are visually more attractive and tasty. In others, the increase in calorie content is mostly due to an increase of lipids. This indicates that specific training for cooks in homes is instrumental in slowing down the progressive decline of intake observed in residents. By inducing higher protein consumption, the improved food quality as a result of the training also helps to reduce a decline in autonomy. Such effects are observed in residents with low BMIs and little appetite – the more fragile residents.

Training on institutional food services in the hospital environment, as a specialist area in the technical field of hotel education, is an important element to raise awareness among cooks and kitchen personnel concerning the impact of appealing and good quality food on the development of undernutrition in older people.[lviii]

Specific recommendations with regard to food provision:

- establish evidence-based recommendations for nutritional quality and quantity of food in care homes and home care food services;
- organise training of kitchen staff to increase their knowledge of the nutritional composition of the food they prepare;
- have the meals and menus composed and controlled by a dietician;
- implement simple tricks and measures to increase the energy and protein content of prepared foods;
- make available energy and protein-rich snacks and supplements between meals;
- have regular controls and audits of food services in care homes and home care.

Home care

Since hospital stays are getting shorter, home care is becoming more important in preventing undernutrition and in continuing nutritional treatment to enable faster social rehabilitation and reintegration, and consequently improving the quality of life. It often is the first level of screening for undernutrition and for identifying high risk factors.

Nevertheless, since a lot of people in home care are dependent on others, suffer from immobility, and psychical and social regression, and are financially restricted, a lot of them also suffer from undernutrition. This is further reinforced by the fact that qualitative and quantitative monitoring of a diet in a domestic context is more complicated, or even impossible, compared to the hospital environment. The family doctor and home care health care workers therefore play a very important role in screening and treatment of undernutrition. In order to carry out this role adequately, they should be sufficiently aware and trained. Unfortunately, as in hospitals, here too ignorance of the problem and its consequences are the main issues, primarily due to a lack of information about the person's condition as recorded in the medical record. This type of information is rarely transmitted among the different care settings (hospitals – care homes – home care services).

Specific recommendations with regard to strategies aimed at tackling undernutrition in home care:

- identification and implementation of the most appropriate and feasible methods for screening and nutritional assessment. Such methods must be simple, easy to use by the caregivers and enable them to identify people at risk or suffering from undernutrition. Those people should then be confided to specialised follow-up by a dietician or the family doctor;
- create a global medical record of each person, describing their nutritional status and personal history in a standard way and make it available to all caregivers. A "nutrition status booklet" may, furthermore, be used for transferring nutritional data about a person's nutritional status in a systematic way between hospitals, home care services and care homes;

- facilitate specialised follow-up. In case of nutritional problems, the person should have access to professional support and follow-up by a dietician. As financial restraints exist that greatly hinder efficient and long-term follow-up, dietetic counselling should be reimbursed. Also, the person's other caregivers should have access to the advice of the dietician and be involved in the nutritional management of the person;
- enable efficient nutritional support as the best and most effective preventive measure to avoid undernutrition. The best way of offering adequate nutritional support is via a normal and balanced diet. In cases where, because of underlying illnesses, lack of enjoyment of food or incapacity, nutritional support in the form of sip and tube feeding is indicated, such support, to be effective in spite of financial constraints, should be reimbursed;
- support home delivery services of grocery foodstuffs and hot meals and facilitate help during eating. In particular, hot meal distribution should be adequately controlled in relation to the nutritional value and properties of the meals. The amount eaten should be recorded or monitored;
- in care homes and hospitals fundamental aspects of nutritional care are included in the overall budget. In the home care situation, most of these aspects have to be paid for additionally, which is a big hindrance to effective nutritional care. It is therefore advisable to financially and structurally support:
  - family and care help for preparing foods and help during eating, in order to avoid the situation where good quality food that is delivered at home is not eaten because of mechanical problems (uncut meat, etc.), dental problems, etc;
  - the provision of affordable food supply and reimbursed supplemental foods, to avoid food not being eaten because it is too expensive or divided over two days, etc;
  - psychological support to avoid alienation;
- develop an awareness-raising campaign on this issue, aimed at health care providers (local GPs, home care organisations, meal delivery organisations, etc.) and at the residents themselves. The goal for the health care providers is to raise their awareness of the recommended simple detection methods, and the description and treatment of

symptoms of undernutrition (clinical impression, information on weight loss, recent illnesses, BMI, etc.). This information can then be used to transfer the person to a local general practitioner or a dietician;

– raise people's awareness through the distribution of a special guide on the topic designed for older people and for non-professional people in charge of their care. Such a guide should elaborate the principles of adequate and balanced nutrition, the necessity of eating properly and sufficient drinking, the need to remain physically active, information on the disadvantages and potential consequences of uncontrolled and restrictive dieting, the importance of proper dental and oral hygiene, the signs that should urge a person to seek specialised advice such as loss of appetite, unexplained weight loss, etc.

The role and responsibilities of society

The person at risk

There is nowadays growing attention to promote more awareness of undernutrition in people themselves, in caregivers and in health care institutions. Attention is paid to adequate information, education, guideline implementation and registration. In the Netherlands, the government has started national improvement programmes for the cure and care sector (improvement programmes of the Ministry of Health, Welfare and Sport (since 2006): Sneller Beter (Cure Faster) and Zorg voor Beter (Care for Better).[lix] In France, educational materials exist in relation to the risk of dehydration during heatwaves.[lx] In Belgium, the National Food and Health Plan foresees educational materials aimed at first-line health professionals, carers and the general population.[iii]

To assess the effectiveness of such measures, the prevalence of undernutrition can become an outcome indicator for the quality of care in all health care settings. In the Netherlands, such initiatives have led to a significant decrease in the prevalence of undernutrition over the last three to four years (see Figure 12).[xix]

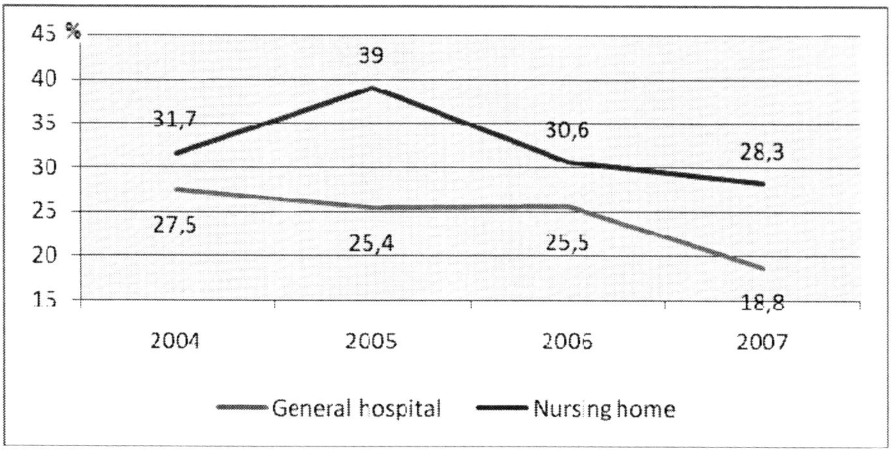

Figure 12: Decline of the prevalence of malnutrition between 2004 and 2007 in the Netherlands[35]

Also, the media and the press have an important role to play in fostering public health messages. This is apparent in relation to smoking and health problems, which feature in many programmes and series. It is less apparent in relation to a balanced diet and the prevention of obesity and undernutrition.

Specific recommendations with regard to awareness and education:

- provide consumer information on healthy and balanced nutrition in a continuous and coherent manner;
- use the most appropriate channels to reach the consumer, for example, audiovisual media, general practitioners, pharmacies, supermarkets, etc;
- create a platform with audiovisual media to enable discussions on the role the media can play to emphasise public health messages (for example, making available advertising space for public health messages, addressing health messages in talk shows, series, etc.);
- address undernutrition with the same attention and means as obesity, and balance messages on the need to eat less to avoid obesity and to eat more to avoid undernutrition.

35. www.faircongress.de/dfc/images/presentations/S1_vanNie_2-5.pdf, p. 15. Date of consultation: November 2008.

Food services

The Council of Europe report highlights food served in many hospitals in the EU is often of poor quality.[2] Hospitals can be expected to serve tasty meals of high nutritional value, which support the patient in their recovery from illness and prevent undernutrition. However, providing appropriate meals at an acceptable cost is often seen as a challenge, when it should not.

The experience of the Centre Hospitalier du Bois de L'Abbaye et de Hesbaye in Seraing, in Belgium, shows how nutritious, healthy, tasty and individually adapted food provision can be achieved using fresh products, purchased through contracts mainly with local producers. Some 910 000 meals are served every year, not only for the associated hospital beds, visitors and staff but also for catering services to people living at home. The Director of Hotel Services, Gerard Filot, works closely together with a team of dieticians and has succeeded, despite the rather limited budgets, to improve the whole experience of eating in the hospital through an emphasis on better service, more varied and attractive menus and fresher, tastier ingredients. The menus are developed in close consultation with the clients (residents, visitors, staff), and include a number of healthy choices in meals. The key factors of success are: bringing nutritional care and food services to the direct attention of the management; continuously monitoring the quality of the catering service; adapting menus and food choices to the needs and preferences of residents; creating a manageable and local supply chain of fresh products; and the training of catering staff to optimise food hygiene and ensure that hazard analysis and critical control point (HACCP) procedures are observed.

Another example is the Schubert balance nutrition concept,[lxi] developed in the early 1990s by the Schubert Group, a Dusseldorf-based service company. This concept is based on the nutritional value guidelines of the German Nutrition Society (DGE) for community catering. In order to comply "daily" with the guidelines of the DGE, the balance concept also includes an electronic data procession (EDP)-supported quality assurance system.

Training and information events are organised in order to convince doctors, nursing staff and kitchen employees of the properties of the balance concept and motivate them to support the concept with respect to the resident. The balance concept is adapted according to a diet catalogue that is based on the latest rationalisation scheme of the German Society of Nutritional Medicine (DGEM). The quality is checked in the form of an annual audit at the respective "balance" facility by the DGE.

The cost of "balance meals" for older individuals at senior citizen facilities is approximately €3.18 a day. This price includes breakfast, lunch, two snacks, an evening meal and drinks.

The balance concept is also implemented in rehabilitation clinics, senior citizen facilities, schools/daycare facilities for children and for people at home by means of "meals on wheels". The basis is the balance concept together with its quality assurance, interfaces with the nursing staff in the home care sector, training of the nursing staff: dietetics/fluid requirements/undernutrition, and information provided to the attending GP. All of this is managed by working groups: nursing staff/doctor/kitchen (diet assistant). The concept offers a balanced lunch with soup and dessert (balance) with options for normal diet, light normal diet, vegetarian and possibly pasta variation and special diets (for example, for diabetics). It includes concepts for undernutrition and swallowing difficulties (for example, thickened liquids). Information material for senior citizens/dependants is provided. Sales prices range from €4.30-6.00 (7% VAT included). It should be noted that the costs of food services may vary considerable between countries (see Figure 13).[lxi]

Average international costs Meals on wheels Source: country-specific suppliers	
Australia	€3.46
Belgium	€5.61
Germany	€5.65
France	€6.08
Austria	€6.24
Italy	€3.75
UK	€5.56
USA	€3.92

Figure 13: National differences in the cost of food services[36]

36. Kohl, O., "Meals in home care: balance between quality and cost", Schubert Unternehmensgruppe, Dusseldorf, Forum on Undernutrition in Care Homes and Home Care. Presentation, November 2007.

In order to guarantee a healthy diet for senior citizens – while remaining within the strict budget – the food is prepared on the basis of a standardised quality assurance system that takes into account scientifically verified nutritional value specifications/guidelines (for example, those of the DGE and the DGEM).

Preparation of food also takes into consideration the special requirements of older individuals, particularly those suffering from dementia.

Interface management between the kitchen, diet assistant, doctor and nursing staff (home care service providers) is essential.

Specific recommendations regarding food services:

- food services should focus on service, varied and attractive menus and fresh, nutritious ingredients, using seasoning with herbs and spices;
- such menus should be developed in close consultation with dieticians to ensure they are nutritionally adequate;
- consultation with the clients (residents, visitors, staff) is important to ensure that the meals and menus correspond to their requirements;
- sufficient choice should be provided, also when addressing specific conditions such as swallowing disorders or medically induced adaptations;
- the management of food service providers should be dedicated to a food quality system and consider all aspects in discussions on what foods to order. Recognition of the importance of appropriate nutrition for reducing undernutrition is vital when considering economic aspects;
- appropriate information and education should be an integral part of food service provision.

Society stakeholders

Educating and informing the public regarding the importance of good nutrition is an essential element in tackling the multifactor causality of undernutrition.

Many society stakeholders are not involved in or aware of the urgent problem of undernutrition. While the EU consumer associations are highly involved in the war against obesity at all levels, they are notably absent in initiatives to tackle undernutrition.

Patients' associations and senior citizens' organisations could play an important role in setting up campaigns to inform people about the importance of nutrition in recovering from an illness. For example, the German organisation Seniorenliga provides interested people with information and educational material. Informed relatives who recognise signs of undernutrition and have knowledge about the related risks are important partners in tackling the issue.[lxii]

Medical professional organisations should evaluate and improve existing professional education programmes, and should keep an eye on the nomination and instalment of the various nutrition managers and committees in the hospitals.

Health insurance funds have an important role to play and some of them have started to address preventive measures with more attention. This leads to a change from "pathology insurance" towards "risk insurance" where screening and scoring are more important than the traditional treatment parameters and where a person can be enrolled into individual care paths and plans. Health care insurance organisations should lobby for a broader reimbursement of nutritional support and also investigate what preventive measures could be taken on their own initiative.

Family help should inform relatives of the dangers of undernutrition and the importance of good nutrition, especially for older people, as well as set up continuous training programmes for their caregivers, focusing on nutrition and how to screen, treat and monitor undernutrition. Finally, meal providers, food services, catering companies and dietary food manufacturers should obtain and provide education on energy-dense menus.

The European Nutrition for Health Alliance, a non-profit alliance of stakeholders, was created in 2005 to raise awareness of the importance and urgency of the undernutrition issue and to put on the agenda at European level. Members include the Association Internationale de la Mutualité (AIM), the European Hospital and Healthcare Federation (HOPE), the European Nursing Directors Association (ENDA), the European Society for Clinical Nutrition and Metabolism (ESPEN), the International Longevity Centre-UK (ILC), the Medical Nutrition International Industry (MNI), the European Union Geriatric Medicine Society (EUGMS) and De Friesland Health Insurance.

On 10 December 2007, a call for action to fight undernutrition in Europe was launched, known as the Prague Declaration.[lxiii] It calls on the EU institutions – the European Parliament, the European Commission and the European Council of Ministers – as well as on national governments, providers of health services and other relevant bodies to:

- acknowledge that undernutrition and obesity are both results of poor nutrition with significant consequences for health outcomes and health care expenditures;
- recognise undernutrition as a distinct pathology and its nutritional support as an integral part of each medical treatment;
- affirm that access to proper nutritional care and support is a fundamental human right;
- offer political direction and support for all stakeholders involved in the fight against undernutrition;
- provide a coherent reimbursement policy for nutritional support across health and social care systems;
- develop nutrition care plans for all health care settings and promote the implementation of existing solutions to fight undernutrition for the benefit of the public, health care systems and society.

Finally, individual projects and research support are also very valuable in raising awareness and mapping out undernutrition and associated aspects. One of those projects is the Nutrition Day in Europe, a large audit which collects information by interviewing people directly about their nutritional care while in hospital, using standardised questionnaires. The project was launched in 2005 by a group of Austrian researchers with the help of a network of national co-ordinators from the European Society of Clinical Nutrition and Metabolism (ESPEN). The aim of Nutrition Day in Europe is to increase awareness and knowledge among people, their caregivers and the public about the importance of nutritional status and care in order to recover from illness. The ultimate goal is to reduce the burden of illness and to decrease health care costs.

In 2006 the audit included 16 455 people from 748 units in 25 countries. The results showed that disease-related undernutrition was associated with a 50% increase in length of stay in hospitals (six days) and is accompanied by a fourfold increase in mortality. The results show the importance of nutritional care and monitoring in health care. The results of the 2006 survey showed that:

- 47% of the respondents had been hospitalised with signs of disease-related undernutrition. Only one out of three people ate all they had been served (38%). One consequence is that the length of stay may increase by 6 days;
- one out of five people ate less than a quarter of what they were offered or nothing at all. Only 11% of those eating very little indicated that they did not like the food. The majority (47%) either had no appetite or had nausea (14%). The reason for this was considered to be the illness itself or the stress of being in hospital;
- reduced appetite is associated with increased mortality. People with an adequate intake had a mortality rate of 1.3%; those with half normal intake, 2.4%; and for all those eating less than a quarter or nothing the rate was more than 5%.

Hospitalised patients with a higher than average body weight had a reduced mortality rate. This apparent advantage is largely negated by the higher risk of becoming ill. Although already this fact was already suspected, the audit confirmed it.

In 2007, for the first time, nursing homes and intensive care units were also able to participate.

Specific recommendations with regard to the role and responsibility of society stakeholders in tackling undernutrition in care homes and home care:

- create national multi-stakeholder platforms to address undernutrition and address contributions and commitments;
- bring the issue of undernutrition to the attention of national and European policy makers;
- address undernutrition in a systematic way as a constant focus point in the stakeholders' action programmes.

The roles and responsibilities of policy makers

In May 2007, the European Commission established a coherent and comprehensive Community strategy to address the issues of overweight and obesity, by adopting the "White Paper on a Strategy for Europe on

Nutrition, Overweight and Obesity-Related Health Issues", focusing on action that can be taken at local, regional, national and European levels to reduce the risks associated with poor nutrition and limited physical exercise, while addressing the issue of inequalities across member states.[lxiv]

This White Paper does not address the equally important issue of undernutrition. At the Forum on Undernutrition in Care Homes and Home Care, organised by the Belgian National Food and Health Plan on 22 and 23 November 2007 in Brussels, Robert Madelin, Director General of DG Sanco, acknowledged that undernutrition was an important issue and explored how it would fit into existing EU health strategies.

On 9 October 2008 the plenary vote on the European Parliament's Health Strategy "Together for Health: Health Strategy 2008-2013" took place.[lxv] During this vote it was unanimously agreed that undernutrition be included as a key target area for policy development and work within the EU over the next five years. The amended strategy gives undernutrition equal weighting with other key public health challenges in Europe including cancer, diabetes, cardiovascular disease, mental health and obesity. The recognition of undernutrition as a major influence on the health of EU citizens is a giant step forward for those working in the field and acknowledges the influence of undernutrition on health and social care as well as on the individual and their carers.

The strategy calls on member states, along with regional and local authorities, to use the co-operation mechanism to improve the exchange of best practice and calls on the Commission to be proactive in producing guidelines and recommendations based on such good practice. As a result, there are now greater opportunities than ever before to tackle the issue of undernutrition in Europe.

With regard to the above-mentioned strategies, national and regional health policy makers, as well as all related policy makers, should make sure that the proper (legislative) frameworks are set in place for the establishment of the necessary working groups and initiatives, so that simple and cost-effective screening methods, treatment plans and monitoring tools can be put in place.

Screening and detecting undernourished people could or should have advantages for the institution. Taking into consideration screening results in the way financial support for care of individual residents is calculated, could be a good approach. The care for and the nutritional support of patients at risk of – or with obvious undernutrition – are obviously greater than for non-undernourished people. However, the increased cost of preventive nutritional support is counterbalanced by the marked economies expected from shorter hospital stays, reduced complications and faster recovery. Providing greater financing for taking responsibility for the nutritional support of undernourished people and reimbursement of supplemental foods are incentives that may encourage institutions to perform systematic screening and help the residents comply with nutritional support by helping them to cope with the extra costs. Special attention should also be given to a coherent reimbursement policy for specialised support and aid by a dietician, and to special food and medically justified dietary products.

Today, although undernutrition represents a significant issue in Europe, requiring urgent action at both EU and member state levels, it is not given the place it deserves on the political agenda. Today's focus is clearly on obesity, while undernutrition and obesity are both results of poor nutrition with significant consequences for health outcomes and health care expenditures. Policy makers must therefore recognise undernutrition as a distinct pathology and its nutritional support as an integral part of each medical treatment.

Specific recommendations with regard to the role and responsibility of policy makers in tackling undernutrition in care homes and home care:

Government policies should:

- assign political responsibility for care of older people. Create a state secretariat for older people;
- develop favourable policies that tackle social isolation, and are in favour of autonomy of older people, intergenerational exchanges and the preservation of autonomy;
- put undernutrition on the political agenda and implement targeted policies; and set standards for nutritional care and support in relation to screening, nutritional assessment and follow-up;
- control and audit compliance with legal and voluntary requirements;
- include screening, assessment and follow-up in the accreditation standards for care homes;
- include nutritional care as an important factor when elaborating criteria for personnel and addressing health care costs;

- provide financial support for expert help by specialised professionals (for example, dieticians) by reimbursing dietetic follow-up and costs for specialised nutrition;
- facilitate systematic transfer of information regarding the nutritional status and nutritional support measures among the different health care settings (hospitals, care homes and home care). Create an interface for regular contact and communication between these settings;
- promote nutritional education in the training of physicians, nurses, caregivers, etc. Education should also focus on multidisciplinary approaches;
- establish minimum standards of education in nutritional support, including agreement on the key functions and responsibilities of the various health care workers. Create possibilities for postgraduate studies and continuous training and education of health care workers leading to a specialisation in nutritional support;
- support initiatives and conduct research on best practices and evidence-based approaches;
- integrate measures to tackle undernutrition as well as obesity and other non-communicable diseases in any national food and health plan.

Conclusions

Undernutrition is defined as a deficiency of energy, protein and other nutrients causing adverse effects on tissue, body form (body shape, size and composition) and function, as well as on clinical outcomes.

The diagnosis of severe undernutrition is based on the presence of one or more of the following criteria: (1) weight loss ≥ 10% in one month or ≥ 15% in six months; (2) BMI < 18 kg/m^2; (3) serum albumin < 30 g/l. Undernutrition is frequent in older individuals living at home (8-19%) and in chronic care institutions (26-38%) according to various European prevalence studies. Older people are at risk of micronutrient deficiency (mainly group B vitamins, vitamin C, vitamin D, selenium, zinc and calcium). Causes that lead to undernutrition include oral and dental disorders, swallowing problems, depression, dementia, chronic diseases, medication, and psychological and social factors associated with loss of autonomy.

Consequences of this state are significant. In particular, undernutrition may prolong the patients' hospital stays, increase the rate of complications by up to 20 times and increase death rates compared to well-nourished patients with the same diseases. Moreover, muscle wasting is also a consequence of undernutrition, which may lead to respiratory failure and physical dependency. Undernutrition can also lead to a state of social isolation and high levels of dependency. Finally, at the level of society, undernutrition-related disease is an economic burden in most countries and preventive medicine should therefore be one of the cornerstones of the actions undertaken to reduce health care costs.

Screening is the first step in assessing and treating undernutrition. The following tools are proposed: (1) Mini Nutritional Assessment (MNA) as the first screening choice; (2) the Malnutrition Universal Screening Tool (MUST) can be second; and (3) Subjective Global Assessment (SGA) is considered as the optimal tool for further nutritional assessment. Screening should be performed on admission to the nursing home and on a regular basis thereafter

A multidisciplinary approach is important in successfully tackling undernutrition at multiple levels: the patients and residents, the health care workers (medical and non-medical), the public, policy makers and society stakeholders. Awareness for people and caregivers is important; this can be achieved by information and appropriate training. Care home management and kitchen staff activities can be modified in order to promote nutrition. Policy makers should create legal frameworks to confront undernutrition as being a public health concern.

A series of recommendation has been proposed in order to act on different levels. With regard to prevalence and causes, recommendations include promoting better nutrition, oral hygiene and avoiding social isolation, as well as encouraging family-style meals in care homes. More specifically for older individuals, it is important to preserve autonomy by offering adapted housing and catering services. Concerning the impact of undernutrition on health care costs, recommendations include enabling smooth transitions from hospital to other settings, expanding reimbursement for dietary counselling, supplemental foods and artificial nutrition. Continuous educational programmes in clinical nutrition may enhance awareness in health care professionals involved in nutritional care of individuals. More specifically, dieticians should have a central role in this domain. Public health messages concerning undernutrition and its consequences must reach all individuals. Finally, government policies should include assigning political responsibility for elderly people and putting undernutrition on the political agenda.

Appendix A: Recommendations of the scientific group of undernutrition experts advising on the Belgian National Food and Health Plan(1): undernutrition screening and nutritional assessment

Introduction

Numerous studies have shown undernutrition to be an independent risk factor that increases the risk of complications, rates of morbidity and mortality, the average length of hospital stays and the overall cost of care.

The prevalence of undernutrition in hospitals, nursing and care homes and primary (community) care varies and depends on the tool used and the population screened. As a rule it varies between 4% and 10% in outpatients, 20% and 62% in hospital inpatients, and 50% and 90% in nursing or care homes. According to the prevalence study conducted in May 2007, which covered more than 80% of Belgium's geriatric units, 35% of those aged over 75 were undernourished and 40% were at imminent risk of undernutrition.[2,3]

The fact that the prognosis for undernourished people improves when they are given adequate nutritional support more than proves the value of screening. But prevention is better than cure. In other words, people at risk of becoming undernourished also need to be identified as quickly as possible.

Screening is the first stage in a two-stage process. All people are screened on admission. If the result is positive, screening must be followed by a more detailed assessment of the individual's nutritional status. This diagnostic procedure is called nutritional assessment. It forms the basis of the nutrition strategy which is drawn up for each person individually.

Screening for undernutrition must be systematically performed by the doctor or nurse when the person is admitted. If the result is positive, a more detailed investigation of the person's nutritional status is essential. This nutritional assessment is more time-consuming than screening and it is performed by a doctor, a dietician or an experienced nurse specialist. The person can also be assessed for his/her risk of undernutrition. If the assessment confirms that the person is undernourished, a nutritional support plan will be drawn up by a dietician, nutrition nurse specialist or the doctor, and the person's dietary intake will be monitored by the nurse or by other care personnel.

This monitoring also includes repeat screening and/or reassessment. This policy is ideally devised and implemented by a multidisciplinary nutrition team.

This document sets out in greater detail the recommendations for screening and nutritional assessment of the adult population (aged 16-18 and over). The group of experts suggests preferred methods for each of the different settings: hospitals, nursing and care homes and primary or home care.

A. Screening for undernutrition

1. Hospitals

Patients are usually placed in an acute unit, either because they are suffering from a condition likely to increase their nutritional requirements or because they need tests or procedures that may mean that their food and fluid intake is markedly reduced. Clearly, the risk of undernutrition for such patients is very real.

Furthermore, rapid turn-over and reduced hospital stay gives nutrition management teams little time to perform screening and if necessary follow it up with nutritional support.

In choosing a screening tool it is important to ensure that it is easy and quick to use and that it can effectively screen all at-risk people.

Nutritional Risk Screening-2002 (NRS-2002)[4] is a method for scoring nutritional risk that consists of a first screening stage (four simple questions) followed by a second stage that assesses the nutritional status or rather the risk of undernutrition. This method has been validated and recognised by ESPEN.[5] For that reason it was selected as the first choice for hospital inpatients.

Its scores take account of the patient's nutritional status and the severity of his/her illness.

See Appendix 1 for a more detailed description.

The Malnutrition Universal Screening Tool (MUST)[6,7,8] is also a valid and effective method. For that reason it was taken as second choice. MUST combines percentage unintentional weight loss, BMI and the acute disease effect. See Appendix 2 for a more detailed description.

Because NRS-2002 is not validated for elderly patients, the group of experts recommends making a distinction between adult patients and patients in a geriatric unit. For the latter group, MUST and the Mini Nutritional Assessment (MNA)[9,10] are the tools of first choice, followed by NRS-2002. MUST and MNA are both equally accurate in identifying the risk of undernutrition in geriatric units.

MUST is easier and more straightforward to use and its questions dovetail more readily with the structure of records kept by nursing staff.

See Appendix 3 for a more detailed description of MNA.

It is important to note that organisational factors within the hospital may have a bearing on which screening tool is ultimately chosen.

Conclusion on screening for undernutrition

Patient	Recommended screening tool	
	1st choice	2nd choice
General (age > 16-18)	NRS-2002	MUST
Elderly patients	MUST or MNA	NRS-2002

2. Nursing and care homes

At present it does not seem that nutritional screening and follow-up are routinely performed even where undernutrition is a recognised problem. Reasons constantly quoted are lack of awareness, time, resources and motivation.

Obviously, a method that is quick and easy will have a better chance of being used. The method must also take account of the population being assessed, namely the elderly.

For these and other reasons, MNA is the first choice for use in this setting. It was developed and validated specifically in elderly people. MUST is the number two choice.

Conclusion on screening for undernutrition

	Recommended screening tool	
	1st choice	2nd choice
All residents	MNA	MUST

3. Primary and home care

As a rule, the health status of outpatients is better than that of people in hospital or care homes. Consequently, where someone comes into contact with a health professional for a reason that is not primarily undernutrition it is important, here more than elsewhere, that the screening tool for undernutrition should be easy and quick to use and of proven efficacy.

The abbreviated form of MNA, MNA-SF (SF = short form),[11] was chosen as the screening tool of choice. MNA-SF constitutes the first part of MNA (Appendix 3, questions A to F).

Bearing in mind that there are also younger people receiving community care, MUST is regarded as better suited to them than MNA-SF.

Conclusion on screening for undernutrition

	Recommended screening tool	
	1st choice	2nd choice
Elderly people	MNA-SF	MUST
Younger people (age > 18)	MUST	

B. Nutritional assessment

Following the initial screening stage, nutritional assessment is required in people who appear, from the screening procedure, to be undernourished. This is a more elaborate procedure than screening and is the basis on which nutrition strategy is built. The nutrition strategy combines medical and nutritional considerations and will ideally be formulated by a multidisciplinary team.

Nutritional assessment is a detailed and structured evaluation of metabolic, nutritional or functional variables designed to identify the person's nutritional status. The assessment is done by a doctor, dietician or nutrition nurse specialist. There are various tools for this: the subjective global assessment, which is primarily clinical, blood tests, muscle strength measured by dynamometry, etc.

None of these is perfect. So a range of methods may be used, though not all of them are clinically very practicable and most of them have a number of disadvantages.

The main method chosen was Subjective Global Assessment (SGA).[12] SGA is a simple, routinely used and proven method for gaining a subjective judgment of the nutritional status. It uses a questionnaire that records the person's medical history and the findings of a physical examination. The most important parameters are percentage weight loss, oedema and a clinical measurement of muscle mass. Professionals prefer SGA because it is simple, practicable and sensitive to virtually the same degree as objective tests.

Dynamometry is very useful but more awkward to perform.

Biochemical parameters such as albumin level are more useful for their predictive value.

> SGA is the most appropriate assessment tool in the different settings. But it is important to realise that SGA can be used as a broad framework and that other aspects have to be taken into account, depending on the person's specific condition.

See Appendix 4 for a more detailed description of SGA.

Conclusions

Screening for undernutrition (Belgian recommendations)

Place	Patient	Recommended screening tool	
		1	2
Hospital	General (adult)	**NRS-2002**	**MUST**
	Elderly patients (age > 75)	**MUST or MNA**	**NRS-2002**
Nursing home/care home	All residents	**MNA**	**MUST**
Community	General (adult)	**MNA-SF**	**MUST**
	Younger people	**MUST**	

Nutritional assessment (Belgian recommendations)

Place	Patient	Recommended nutritional assessment tool
Hospital	General (adult)	**SGA**
	Elderly patients	**SGA**
Nursing home/care home	All residents	**SGA**
Community	General (adult)	**SGA**
	Younger people	**SGA**

It is possible to adapt the implementation of an appropriate method of nutritional screening and assessment to the organisation of any institution or ward; what matters is that screening exists and that a workable nutritional management strategy is implemented in everyday practice.

The components of nutrition strategy are set out in Appendix 5.

References

1. SPF Santé Publique, Securité de la Chaine Alimentaire et Environnement, Plan National Nutrition Santé pour la Belgique, www.monplannutrition.be.

2. SPF Santé Publique, Securité de la Chaine Alimentaire et Environnement, Stratégie pour l'Approche transmurale de la problématique alimentaire chez les personnes âgées, 2006, www.ebnursing.ugent.be/richtlijnen/voeding.

3. Defloor, T., Grypdonck, M., Bocquaert, I., Vanderwee, K., Lardennois, M. and Folens, B., "Evaluation de la dénutrition dans les unites de gériatrie", SPF Santé Publique, Securité de la Chaine Alimentaire et Environnement, 2007.

4. Nutritional Risk Screening-2002 (NRS-2002), Kondrup, J., Rasmussen, H., Hamberg, O. and Stanga, Z., Ad hoc ESPEN Working Group, "Nutritional risk screening (NRS 2002): a new method based on an analysis of controlled clinical trials", *Clinical Nutrition*, 22 (3), June 2003, pp. 321-336.

5. Kondrup, J., Allison, S.P., Elia, M., Vellas, B. and Plauth, M., "ESPEN Guidelines for Nutrition Screening, 2002", *Clinical Nutrition*, 22 (4), 2003, pp. 415-421.

6. MUST: Malnutrition Universal Screening Tool, BAPEN Nutrition Advisory Group, www.bapen.org.uk/must_tool.html.

7. Stratton, R.J., Hackston, A., Longmore, D. et al., "Malnutrition in hospital outpatients and inpatients: prevalence, concurrent validity and ease of use of the 'malnutrition universal screening tool' ('MUST') for adults", *British Journal of Nutrition*, 92 (5), 2004, pp. 799-808.

8. Stratton, R.J., King, C.L., Stroud, M.A., Jackson, A.A. and Elia, M., "'Malnutrition Universal Screening Tool' predicts mortality and length of hospital stay in acutely ill elderly", *British Journal of Nutrition*, 95 (2), 2006, pp. 325-330.

9. MNA: Mini Nutritional Assessment, Guigoz, Y., Vellas, B. and Garry, P.J., "Mini nutritional assessment: a practical assessment tool for grading the nutritional state of elderly patients", *Facts, Res Gerontol (suppl. nutrition)*, second edition, 1994, pp. 15-59, www.mna-elderly.com.

10. Vellas, B., Villars, H., Abellan, G. et al., "Overview of the MNA – Its history and challenges", *Journal of Nutrition, Health and Ageing*, 10 (6), 2006, pp. 456-463, discussion 63-5.

11. MNA-SF: Mini Nutritional Assessment – Short Form.

12. SGA: Subjective Global Assessment, Detsky, A.S., Mclaughin, J.R. and Baker, J.P., "What is subjective global assessment of nutritional status?", *JPEN*, 11 (8), 1987.

Appendices

Appendix 1: Nutritional Risk Screening-2002 (NRS-2002)

Appendix 2: Malnutrition Universal Screening Tool (MUST)

Appendix 3: Mini Nutritional Assessment (MNA) + MNA-SF (questions A to F)

Appendix 4: Subjective Global Assessment (SGA)

Appendix 5: Components of nutrition strategy

Appendix 1: Nutritional Risk Screening-2002 (NRS-2002)

Table 1: Initial screening

		Yes	No
1	Is BMI < 20.5?		
2	Has the patient lost weight within the last three months?		
3	Has the patient had a reduced dietary intake in the last week?		
4	Is the patient severely ill (for example, in intensive therapy) ?		

Yes: If the answer is "Yes" to any question, the screening in Table 2 is performed.
No: If the answer is "No" to all questions, the patient is re-screened at weekly intervals. If the patient, for example, is scheduled for a major operation, a preventive nutritional care plan is considered to avoid the associated risk status.

Table 2: Final screening (nutritional risk assessment)

Impaired nutritional status		Severity of disease (increase in requirements)	
Absent: Score 0	Normal nutritional status	Absent: Score 0	Normal nutritional requirements
Mild: Score 1	Weight loss > 5% in three months or food intake below 50-75% of normal requirement in preceding week	Mild: Score 1	Hip fracture – chronic patients, in particular with acute complications: cirrhosis, COPD, chronic haemodialysis, diabetes, oncology
Moderate: Score 2	Weight loss > 5% in two months or BMI = 18.5-20.5 + impaired general condition or food intake 25-60% of normal requirement in preceding week	Moderate: Score 2	Major abdominal surgery, stroke, severe pneumonia, haematologic malignancy
Severe: Score 3	Weight loss > 5% in one month (> 15% in three months) or BMI < 18.5 + impaired general condition or food intake 0-25% of normal requirement in preceding week	Severe: Score 3	Head injury, bone marrow transplantation, intensive care patients (APACHE > 10)
Score:	+	score:	= total score
Age: if ≥ 70, add 1 to total score above = age-adjusted total score			
Score ≥ 3: the patient is nutritionally at risk and a nutritional care plan is initiated. Score < 3: weekly re-screening of the patient. If the patient is, for example, scheduled for a major operation, a preventive nutritional care plan is considered to avoid the associated risk status.			

Appendix 2: Malnutrition Universal Screening Tool (MUST)

Step 1 BMI score	+	Step 2 Weight loss score	+	Step 3 Acute disease effect score
BMI (kg/m^2) Score > 20 (> 30 = obese) = 0 18.5-20 = 1 < 18.5 = 2		Unplanned weight loss in past three to six months Score < 5% = 0 5-10% = 1 > 10% = 2		If the patient is acutely ill and there has been or is likely to be no nutritional intake for > five days Score = 2

If unable to obtain height and weight, alternative measurements including subjective criteria may be used.

Step 4
Overall risk of malnutrition

Add scores together to calculate overall risk of malnutrition

Score 0	Score 1	Score 2 or more
Low risk	Medium risk	High risk

Step 5
Management guidelines

0 Low risk Routine clinical care	1 Medium risk Observe	2 or more High risk Treat*
Repeat screening Hospital – weekly Care home – monthly Community – annually for special groups, for example, those >75	Hospital – document dietary and fluid intake for three days if subject in hospital or care home	Refer to dietician or nutritional support team, or implement local policy
	If improved or adequate intake – little clinical concern If no improvement – clinical concern – follow local policy	Improve and increase overall nutritional intake
	Repeat screening Hospital – weekly Care homes – monthly Community – at least every two to three months	Monitor and review care plan Hospital – weekly Care home – monthly Community – monthly
		*Unless detrimental or no benefit is expected from nutritional support, for example, imminent death.

All risk categories:	**Obesity:**
Treat underlying condition and provide help and advice on food choices, eating and drinking when necessary Record malnutrition risk category Record need for special diets and follow local policy	Record presence of obesity For those with underlying conditions, these are generally controlled before the treatment of obesity

Reassess subjects identified at risk as they move through care settings (hospital, care home, community)

Appendix 3: Mini Nutritional Assessment (MNA) + MNA-SF (questions A to F)

Last name: First name: Sex: Date:
Age: Weight (kg): Height (cm): Knee height (cm):
Complete the screen by filling in the boxes with the appropriate numbers.
Add the numbers for the screen.
If score is 11 or less, continue with the assessment to gain a Malnutrition Indicator Score.

Screening

A	Has food intake declined over the past three months due to loss of appetite, digestive problems, chewing or swallowing difficulties? 0 = severe loss of appetite 1 = moderate loss of appetite 2 = no loss of appetite	Score
B	Weight loss during last three months 0 = weight loss > 3 kg 1 = does not know 2 = weight loss between 1 and 3 kg 3 = no weight loss	Score
C	Mobility 0 = bed or chair bound 1 = able to get out of bed/chair but does not go out 2 = goes out	Score
D	Has suffered physical stress or acute disease in the past 3 months 0 = yes 2 = no	Score
E	Neuropsychological problems 0 = severe dementia or depression 1 = mild dementia 2 = no psychological problems	Score

J	How many full meals does the patient eat daily? 0 = 1 meal 1 = 2 meals 2 = 3 meals		Score
K	Selected consumption markers for protein intake:		
	At least one serving of dairy products (milk, cheese, yogurt) per day	yes	no
	Two or more servings of vegetables or eggs per week	yes	no
	Meat, fish or poultry every day	yes	no
	0.0 = if 0 or 1 yes 0.5 = if 2 yes 1.0 = if 3 yes		Score
I	Consumes two or more servings of fruit or vegetables per day? 0 = no 1 = yes		Score
M	How much fluid (water, juice, coffee, tea, milk, wine, beer ...) is consumed per day? 0.0 = less than 3 cups 0.5 = 3 to 5 cups 1.0 = more than 5 cups		Score
N	Mode of feeding 0 = unable to eat without assistance 1 = self-fed with some difficulty 2 = self-fed without any problem		Score

F	Body Mass Index (BMI = weight/(height in m)^2 0 = BMI < 19 1 = 19 ≤ BMI < 21 2 = 21 ≤ BMI < 23 3 = BMI ≥ 23	Score

Screening score (subtotal, maximum 14 points):

12 points or greater	Normal – not at risk → no need to complete assessment
11 points or below	Possible malnutrition → continue assessment

Assessment

G	Lives independently (not in a nursing home or hospital) 0 = no 1 = yes	Score
H	Takes more than three prescription drugs per day 0 = yes 1 = no	
I	Pressure sores or skin ulcers 0 = yes 1 = no	Score

References: Vellas, B., Villars, H., Abellan, G., et al., "Overview of the MNA – Its history and challenges", *Journal of Nutrition, Health and Ageing*, 10 (6), 2006, pp. 456-465.

Rubenstein, L.Z., Harker, J.O., Salva, A., Guigoz, Y. and Vellas, B., "Screening for malnutrition in geriatric practice: developing the Short-Form Mini Nutritional Assessment (MNA-SF)", *Journal of Gerontology*, 56A, 2001, pp. M366-377.

Guigoz, Y., "The Mini Nutritional Assessment (MNA). Review of the Literature – What does it tell us?", *Journal of Nutrition, Health and Ageing*, 10, 2006, pp. 466-487.

Nestlé, 1994, revision 2006

O	Self view of nutritional status 0 = views self as being malnourished 1 = is uncertain of nutritional state or views self as moderately malnourished 2 = views self as having no nutritional problem	Score
P	In comparison with other people of the same age, how does the patient consider his/her health status? 0.0 = not as good 0.5 = does not know 1.0 = as good 2.0 = better	Score
Q	Mid-arm circumference (MAC) in cm 0.0 = MAC < 21 0.5 = ≥ 21 MAC ≤ 22 1.0 = MAC > 22	Score
R	Calf circumference (CC) in cm 0 = CC < 31 1 = CC ≥ 31	Score

Assessment (maximum 16 points)
Screening score (maximum 14 points)
Total assessment (maximum 30 points)

Malnutrition Indicator Score

17 to 23.5 points	at risk of malnutrition
Less than 17 points	malnourished

Appendix 4: Subjective Global Assessment (SGA)

Item	Interpretation	Score
Weight loss (3-6 months)	Automatically (= question in initial screening)	Score 0 = A Score 1 = B Score 2 or 3 = C
Pattern of weight loss (3-6 months)	5-10% continuous loss 5-10% loss, but improvement > 10% continuous loss > 10% loss, but continuous improvement	B A C B
Muscle wasting	Little or no loss in most or all body locations Mild to moderate loss in most or all body locations Moderate to severe loss in some body locations Severe loss in most or all body locations	A B B C
Oedema	Little or none Mild to moderate Moderate to severe	A B C
Subcutaneous fat loss	Little or no loss in most or all body locations Mild to moderate loss in most or all body locations Moderate to severe loss in some body locations Severe loss in most or all body locations	A B B C
Change in dietary intake	No change or short-lived change Reduced intake but improvement Reduced intake but deterioration	A B C
Duration of change in dietary intake	< two weeks > two weeks, nourishment mildly to moderately inadequate Unable to eat	A B C
Gastrointestinal symptoms	No or few symptoms Moderate symptoms > two weeks Severe symptoms but improvement Symptom(s) > two weeks	A B B C
Functional impairment	No change Severe loss but improvement Bedridden	A B C

Number of A ratings:	A: well nourished
Number of B ratings:	B: mild/moderate malnutrition
Number of C ratings:	C: severe malnutrition

Appendix 5: Components of nutrition strategy

	1. Screening for undernutrition and risk of undernutrition
NRS-2002 MUST MNA	1a. Screening for undernutrition and risk of undernutrition BMI Degree of recent weight loss Food intake Illness(es)
	2. Nutritional assessment
SGA	2a. Medical history Causes of weight loss Food habits Changes in food intake Drugs Gastrointestinal symptoms/function Increased requirements
SGA	2b. Physical examination Muscle mass/stores of subcutaneous fat Examination/palpation to detect oedema/ascites Signs/symptoms of vitamin/mineral deficiency
Other nutritional assessment parameters that may be used	2c. Function tests Example: hand dynamometry
Other nutritional assessment parameters that may be used	2d. Biochemical parameters Long-term: albumin Short-term: prealbumin and transferrin
	3. Nutritional management
Nutritional management	3a. Assessment of dietary intake and nutritional requirements Dietary intake: current situation, prediction of improvement/deterioration Indirect calorimetry
Nutritional care plan devised by the nutrition team	3b. Nutritional management Type of feeding (enteral/parenteral, complete/complementary, supplements, etc.)
Patient medical file – nutrition record booklet	3c. Recording and transfer of data Transfer of data between hospital – nursing/care home – community/home care and monitoring

Components of nutrition strategy

Undernutrition is managed in three stages, of which screening is the first. All people are screened systematically on admission. If the result is positive, screening must be followed by a more detailed assessment of the person's nutritional status (nutritional assessment). If this confirms that the person is undernourished, a nutritional care plan will be drawn up based on assessment of the person's dietary intake and nutritional requirements. The undernourished person will be monitored by a dietician and the doctor, and nutritional support will be initiated.

1. Screening

Screening is a method for assessing the person's risk of undernutrition. Body Mass Index (BMI), recent weight loss, dietary intake and the person's illness or other medical conditions are taken into account in this assessment.

In choosing a screening tool it is important to ensure that it is easy and quick to use by non-specialist personnel (care team) and that it can screen all at-risk persons. The most appropriate method will vary with the circumstances (hospital, care home or home care). A summary of the methods best suited to each situation has been prepared by the Scientific Group of Undernutrition Experts advising on Belgium's National Food and Health Plan (NFHP-B):

Place	Patient	Recommended screening tool	
		1st	2nd
Hospital	General (adult)	**NRS-2002**	**MUST**
	Geriatric unit	**MUST or MNA**	**NRS-2002**
Nursing home/care home	All residents	**MNA**	**MUST**
Community (patient's own home)	General (adult)	**MNA-SF**	**MUST**
	Younger people	**MUST**	

When screening suggests that the person is undernourished or at increased risk of undernutrition, the doctor is notified, the person is referred to a dietician for nutritional assessment and assessment of food intake and to initiate a nutritional care strategy.

2. Nutritional assessment

Nutritional assessment is performed on people whose screening result is positive. This assessment forms the basis of the nutrition strategy which is drawn up for each person individually. It is more time-consuming than screening and it is performed by a doctor, a dietician or an experienced nurse specialist. This assessment consists of the following:

2.a. Medical history

The person's medical history is the starting point for nutritional management. This will reveal the following factors: any causes of a recent weight loss, dietary habits and any changes in them, drugs that may affect appetite, any drug-nutrient interactions, gastrointestinal function and symptoms, any increased requirement for micro- or macronutrients, current functional capacity and the person's pre-admission state of health.

2.b. Physical examination

One of the main reasons for physically examining the person is to ascertain whether he/she has any dietary insufficiency and whether nutritional support is well tolerated.

The physical examination must include at least:

- an estimate of muscle mass and stores of subcutaneous fat;
- examination and palpation to detect oedema and ascites
- signs and symptoms of vitamin and mineral deficiency.

Aspects 2.a and 2.b are the basic components of the Subjective Global Assessment (SGA). The SGA is the assessment tool of choice in the different settings (hospital, care home, community).

2.c. Function tests

Function tests such as dynamometry are useful but are often awkward to perform and unnecessary.

Hand dynamometry is one example of a function test. Maximum handgrip strength is an indication of peripheral muscle function and relates to total muscle mass. A decrease in hand muscle strength may be a sign of muscle loss.

2.d. Biochemical parameters

Biochemical parameters are not necessary either. They are more valuable as predictors. A number of biochemical parameters may be used (serum proteins, vitamins and minerals, etc.). Some of them can be used to assess nutritional status and to monitor the efficacy of nutritional support. Serum proteins have a different half-life. Serum albumin is a good predictor of disease outcome and seriousness. It is a poor marker of nutritional status, however, though it can be useful for long-term monitoring. For short-term monitoring, prealbumin and transferrin are more useful.

3. Management of the undernourished person

If nutritional assessment confirms that the person is undernourished, appropriate nutritional support is initiated, based on assessment of the person's dietary intake and nutritional requirements.

3.a. Assessment of dietary intake and energy and nutritional requirements

Assessing dietary intake and comparing this with nutritional requirements not only provides a snapshot of the person's current status; it also helps to predict how the person's nutritional status is likely to improve or deteriorate. Accurate estimation of dietary intake is a real challenge. Given the fact of day-by-day variability, intake is assessed over several days. The method used to do this will depend on the person's situation: dietary intake record using the twenty-four-hour recall method, kept over a full week by the dietician, food diary completed by the person, or dietary consumption sheets completed by the staff looking after the person. These data can subsequently be used by the dietician to calculate dietary intake in terms of energy, proteins, lipids, carbohydrates, minerals, vitamins and water.

Energy requirement may be measured (using indirect calorimetry) or estimated using formulae. Nutritional recommendations for various nutrients are detailed in the literature and should be used to optimise dietetic advice.

3.b. Nutritional management

Nutritional management of the undernourished person is overseen by a dietician and the doctor, based on assessment of the dietary intake, nutritional requirement and the person's medical condition. Psychosocial factors are also taken into account.

Appropriate nutritional support may entail adaptation of the normal diet or the use of specialist dietetic foods, including foods delivered enterally by nasogastric or gastrostomy tube or parenterally, complete or complementary foods or specific nutritional supplements, which may or may not be tailored to the person's medical condition. Nutritional care plans may be drawn up.

Help with feeding, dental care and adequate fluid intake are other factors to be borne in mind.

3.c. Monitoring of nutritional support

From food and fluid intake record sheets or a food diary, the person's nutritional status can be monitored and the efficacy of support assessed. Monitoring of weight and biochemical parameters provide meaningful indications only over a longer period of time.

3.d. Recording and transfer of data

The person's data, collected in the course of screening, nutritional assessment and nutritional management, must be placed in his/her medical file and must travel with the person between one level of care and another (hospital, care home, home care).

A "nutrition record booklet" or similar document may be useful here.

Appendix B: Practical measures set out in the "nutrition quality charter" for care homes (CHs) and care and nursing homes (CNHs)

Criteria for the certification of care homes that have been awarded the regional "nutrition quality" label, to be taken into account in community, regional and federal legislation

Introduction to the charter

The Belgian National Food and Health Plan (NFHP-B) recognises that many elderly people suffer from undernutrition.

Although food is usually provided in sufficient quantity and quality in care and nursing homes and other residential facilities for the elderly, it has been found that a significant percentage of residents are undernourished. Proper nutrition, however, is essential for maintaining health, ensuring rapid recovery and building resistance, and for well-being in general.

The problem of undernutrition stems mainly from lack of regulation, not only of the quantity and quality of the meals served but also of the monitoring of residents' nutritional status. This is compounded by the lack of structural support for a food policy in institutions, including staff qualifications.

Under the NFHP-B operational plan, a working group was tasked with drawing up a nutritional charter. Institutions that implement it would be awarded a "nutrition quality" label and the charter would be enshrined in law at community, regional and federal level.

This charter has now been completed and is available on the NFHP-B website. Public services in the Walloon Region have undertaken to road-test the charter while the working group is to continue its activities by looking at the costs and workload for institutions.

Content

Practical measures set out in the "nutrition quality charter" for care homes (CHs) and care and nursing homes (CNHs)

Criteria for the certification of care homes that have been awarded the regional "nutrition quality" label, to be taken into account in community, regional and federal legislation.

A. Establishing procedures for screening and assessing the nutritional status of elderly people[37]

The aim is to detect undernutrition and assess the nutritional status of elderly people by means of simple, rapid and practical tools that are easy and inexpensive to use.

Prerequisites

The detection and monitoring of undernutrition in CHs/CNHs must be part of the overall assessment of elderly people's state of health and the corresponding corrective measures. It is particularly important to check weight and dental and oral hygiene regularly and, at all events, at least one a month.

Recording weight on an individual chart[38] will help to trigger an alarm when there is an abnormal change in weight.

In order to do this there must be sufficient staff.

Screening: MNA

There are several methods for detecting undernutrition. The Scientific Group of Experts on Undernutrition (PNNS-B) has recommended the most appropriate methods for screening for undernutrition. In the case of elderly people living in care homes, the method used is the Mini Nutritional Assessment (MNA).

The nutritional status of the elderly person is systematically assessed by means of the MNA in five different circumstances:

- on admission;

37. Based on the conclusions of the group of experts on screening for undernutrition and nutritional assessment.
38. Graphic chart

- in the event of weight loss of > 2% in one week, > 5% in one month and > 10% in six months;
- once a month;
- on prescription;
- on discharge or transfer to another establishment.

The person's height is measured on admission and at least once a year (using a height gauge or laser).

If the MNA suggests that there is a risk of undernutrition, the nutritional assessment is made according to the Subjective Global Assessment (SGA) method, by a doctor, a dietician, or a nurse who has taken a specialised training course in nutrition.

This means that elderly people cared for in residential establishments should:

- either have an MNA that has been carried out at least within the previous thirty-one days, indicating that their nutritional status is normal; or
- be undergoing a nutritional care programme.

Irrespective of whether or not they are receiving nutritional care, elderly people must be weighed once a week.

The MNA can be carried out by a nurse, a nurse aid, a dietician or a doctor.

This method is summarised in the flow chart in Appendix 1.

Nutritional assessment: SGA

Depending on the results of the screening test, it may be necessary to assess the nutritional status of people whose test suggests that there is risk of undernutrition.

Subjective Global Assessment (SGA) is a frequently used and approved method of assessing a person's nutritional status. The method consists of a questionnaire on the person's background and a clinical examination. Professionals prefer SGA because it is a simple, practical and sensitive method and almost comparable to objective tests.

The SGA is carried out by a doctor, a dietician or a nurse who has received training in nutrition as they have the necessary expertise in this field.

This method is summarised in the flow chart in Appendix 1.

B. Ensuring that a member of staff is responsible for food quality and nutrition

- with a degree in food nutrition;
- in each establishment (FTE (full-time equivalent) proportionate to the number of residents);
- ensures that the charter is correctly applied;
- ensures the quality of food and meals;
- supervises food hygiene;
- helps plan menus and meals;
- helps purchase food and food supplements;
- is in charge of supervising the individual nutrition of each resident together with his/her doctor or the co-ordinating doctor and the medical team.

C. Establishing a food and nutrition liaison committee

- comprising professional staff involved in nutrition (cook, dietician, medical staff, logotherapist, physiotherapist, ergonomist, etc.);[39]
- working for one (CHs/CNHs > 70 elderly people) or several establishments, with the approval of the certifying body;
- to guarantee the flow of information on the nutritional status and treatment of the elderly person among all those concerned (internal and external);
- to establish procedures with regard to screening for undernutrition and supervising undernourished people;
- to formulate appropriate food therapies tailored to the different situations and conditions;
- to draw the attention of the entire staff to the problem of undernutrition and arrange for appropriate in-service training.

---

39. Given the large number of professionals involved in nutrition, it is essential (in practice) that at least three of the following professionals – doctor, nurse, dietician, cook, representative of the management – be present so that decisions can be taken and implemented.

D. Creating a pleasant environment and a suitable atmosphere during meals

Minimum criteria:

- pleasant, friendly setting;
- sufficient staff should be present at each meal to assist the elderly people;[40]
- appropriate equipment should be available to help elderly people eat and drink;
- elderly people should be allowed to give their opinion on the quality of the meals and menus served and their opinion should be taken into account by the "board of residents" and the person responsible for food quality and nutrition.

E. Guaranteeing access to a healthy and balanced diet

Minimum criteria:

- offer a sufficiently wide choice;[41]
- respect elderly people's dietary habits and preferences;
- provide individual food rations suited to the elderly person's tastes and preferences to ensure that each elderly person has an appropriate intake of food;
- propose menus and meals (according to the principles set out in the National Food and Health Plan) drawn up and approved by a dietician.

F. Qualified and properly trained staff

Minimum criteria:

- cooks in care homes should have a qualification in mass catering;[42]
- there should be a specific training programme for staff working with senior citizens and refresher courses (in-service training) for all staff

---

40. This criterion is of prime importance as it is the weakest link in the chain: if the person concerned does not have the possibility to eat, the charter is doomed to failure. Although it may be impossible to increase the number of staff, the management can be obliged to ensure that all staff on duty are present during meals and to deploy staff on duty during the day, at weekends and during public holidays so that there are always sufficient staff present at meals.

41. There must be a wide enough choice and range of food offered at meals. Minimum: one breakfast, one lunch, a choice of two evening meals and a choices of two snacks.

42. Existing staff should be offered the opportunity to take a refresher course in mass catering for elderly people.

working in care homes, concerning the specific problem of the undernutrition of elderly people.

G. Exchange of information between hospitals, CHs/CNHs and home care with a view to improving dietary supervision in the form of a medical and nutritional file (nutritional record booklet) for each elderly person

Comments:

- The earlier undernutrition is diagnosed the more effective the treatment, which means that it is important to target not only CNHs but also CHs where elderly people are, in theory, less dependent.
- Physical exercise is a decisive factor for the good health of people of all ages and plays an important role in preventing and treating undernutrition; as it has an impact on bones and muscles reducing the processes of osteolysis and sarcopenia associated with ageing. In order to comply with the charter, it is also necessary to establish a programme of physical activities suited to the physical condition of the elderly people concerned.
- The amendment of the Royal Decree of 21 September 2004 stipulating the requirements for certification as a care and nursing home or as a daycare centre, in particular the organisational guidelines set out in Appendix I relating to care and nursing homes, must be presented as a long-term goal as the principle of the charter is that residential establishments should be free to adopt it, independently of compulsory requirements.

Appendix 1: Screening flow chart

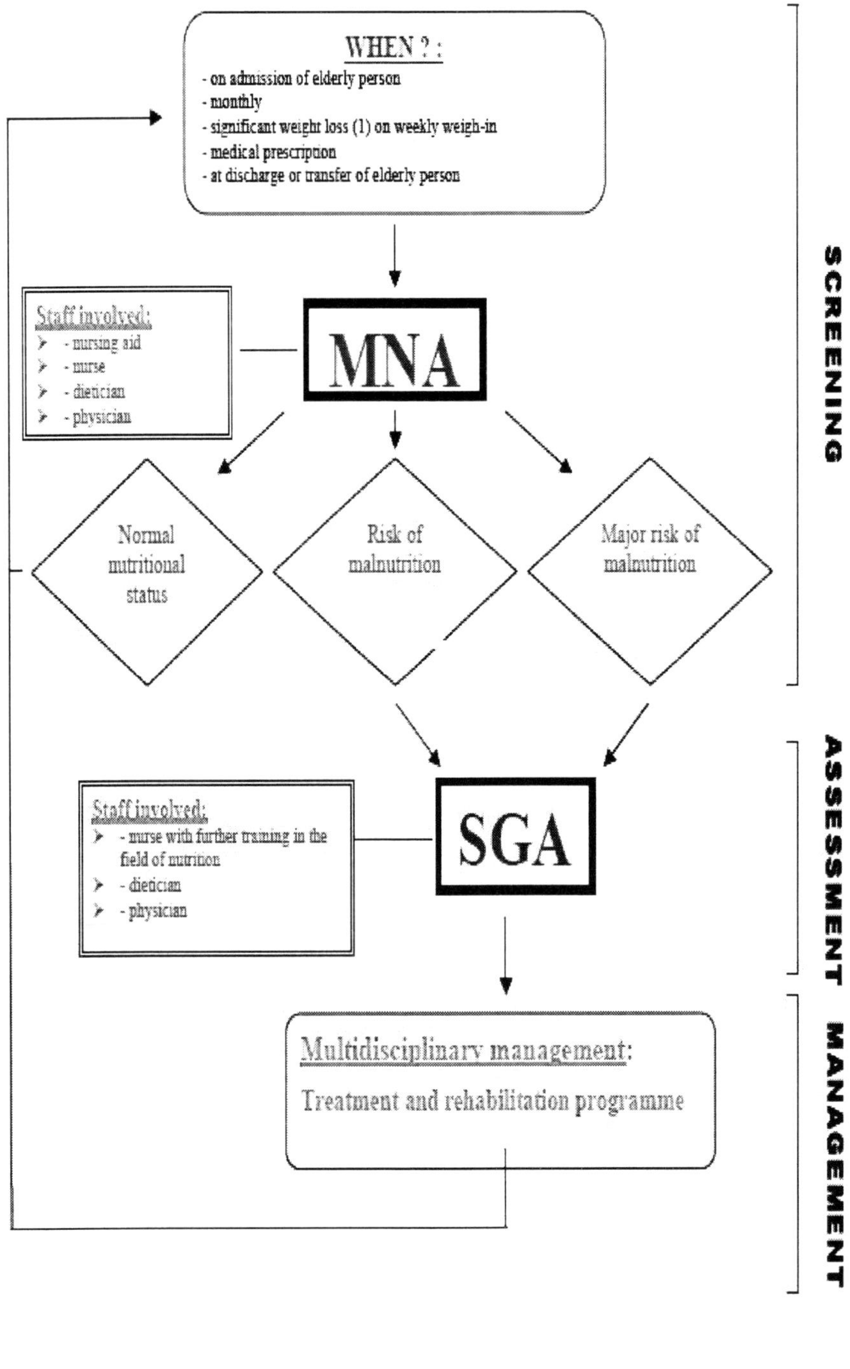

Appendix 2: Tasks of dieticians in preventing undernutrition[43] in elderly people in care homes

- seeing to the quality and variety of meals on offer;
- analysing menus, participating in the formulation of recipes and suggesting alternatives in co-ordination with the cook and the purchasing officer;
- seeing to a wider choice of menus at each meal and organising choices with the cook (planning ahead);
- agreeing food purchases with the cook and the purchasing officer;
- checking and adapting food rations to ensure that each elderly person has an appropriate intake of food;
- attending meetings of the board of residents;
- joining with the management and the cook in assessing resident satisfaction on the basis of the opinions of the board of residents;
- participating in food hygiene assessment and corrective measures together with the kitchen staff, nurses and external bodies mandated for this purpose (Food Safety Agency – hygiene food inspection);
- participating on a multidisciplinary basis in the nutritional monitoring of all residents;
- setting up, participating in and assessing screening for undernutrition (see attached flow chart);
- meeting regularly with the doctor and nurse of the care home to review dietetic measures for undernourished residents;
- joining with the doctor in formulating appropriate food therapies tailored to the different situations and conditions;
- participating in meals and, if necessary, helping residents;
- maintaining regular contact with each resident to ensure personalised nutritional intake.

---

43. Dieticians working in care homes obviously fit their work in with the plan as a whole, as well as with all the other activities associated with their area of expertise: prevention of obesity, diets tailored to medical conditions other than undernutrition, etc. The duties detailed above are therefore not an exhaustive list of the duties of a dietician working in a care home. They must be regarded as additional services, whose extent will depend on how the institution is organised and the experience, knowledge and competence of all the staff. If the dietician is regarded as the key figure in establishing all the activities falling within the scope of the charter, that should be taken into account in his or her overall workload.

Within the food and nutrition liaison committee

- sitting on and leading the food and nutrition liaison committee. Any collective initiative in support of the charter must be approved by the committee and the management;
- suggesting to the management, all the staff and the residents any suitable measures for implementing the charter in the care home;
- making arrangements with the doctor to ensure that residents' nutrition files are circulated among the nursing and care staff of the care home and are made available for primary care consultations;
- introducing measures for raising awareness of the plan and suggesting training for the staff involved;
- participating in decisions relating to the setting or environment in which meals are taken;
- ensuring, together with the management, that sufficient staff are deployed at mealtimes;
- participating in the recruitment of staff concerned with food and nutrition.

NFHP-B, August 2008

Bibliography

i. Council of Europe, *Food and nutritional care in hospitals: how to prevent undernutrition*, report and recommendations of the Committee of Experts on Nutrition, Food Safety and Consumer Protection, Council of Europe Publishing, Strasbourg, 2003.

ii. Council of Europe Committee of Ministers Resolution ResAP(2003)3 on food and nutritional care in hospitals, 2003.

iii. Belgian Ministry of Social Affairs and Public Health, "National Food and Health Plan for Belgium 2005-2010", FOD Volksgezondheid, Veiligheid van de Voedselketen en Leefmilieu, Brussels, 2007. https://portal.health.fgov.be/pls/portal/docs/page/internet_pg/homepage_menu/mijngezondheid1_menu/produitsdeconsommation1_menu/alimentation1_menu/plannutritionsante1_menu/infopourprofessionnels1_menu/infopourprofessionnels1_docs/pnns-b%20def.pdf. Date of consultation: 27 October 2008.

iv. Arvanitakis, M. et al., "Nutrition in care homes and home care: how to implement adequate strategies (report of the Brussels Forum (22 to 23 November 2007))", *Clinical Nutrition*, 27, 2008, pp. 481-488. https://portal.health.fgov.be/pls/portal/docs/page/internet_pg/homepage_menu/mijngezondheid1_menu/produitsdeconsommation1_menu/alimentation1_menu/belgique1_menu/denutritiondansleshopitauxmaisonsde_hide/denutritiondansleshopitauxmaisonsde_docs/nutrition%20in%20care%20homes%20and%20home%20care.pdf. Date of consultation: 27 October 2008.

v. Heyneman, A. et al., *Strategie voor de transmurale aanpak van de voedingsproblematiek bij ouderen*, Federale Overheidsdienst Volksgezondheid, Veiligheid van de Voedselketen en Leefmilieu, Brussels, 2006.

vi. Defloor, T. et al., *Evaluatie van ondervoeding binnen geriatrische afdelingen*, FOD Volksgezondheid, Veiligheid van de Voedselketen en Leefmilieu, Brussels, 2007.

vii. Stratton, R.J., Green, C.J. and Elia, M., *Disease-related malnutrition: an evidence-based approach to treatment*. Wallingford: CABI; 2003

viii. Haute Autorité de Santé, "Stratégie de prise en charge en cas de dénutrition protéino-énergétique chez la personne âgée", Haute Autorité de Santé, Service communication, Saint-Denis La Plaine, 2007. www.has-sante.fr/portail/upload/docs/application/pdf/denutrition_personne_agee_2007_-_recommandations.pdf. Date of consultation: 27 October 2008.

ix. Ribbe, M.W., Ljunggren, G., Steel, K., Topinkova, E., Hawes, C., Ikegami, N., Henrard, J.C. and Jonnson, P.V., "Nursing homes in 10 nations: a comparison between countries and settings", *Age and Ageing*, 26-S2, 1997, pp. 3-12.

x. Bourdel-Marchasson, I. et al., "Undernutrition in geriatric institutions in South-West France: policies and risk actors", *Nutrition*, published electronically ahead of print, 8 October 2008.

xi. www.lpz-um.nl. Date of consultation: 27 October 2008.

xii. Meijers, J.M. et al., "Malnutrition prevalence in the Netherlands: results of the Annual Dutch National Prevalence Measurement of Care Problems", *Br J Nutr*, pp. 1-7, published electronically ahead of print, 5 June 2008.

xiii. "Landelijke Prevalentiemeting Zorgproblemen. Rapportage resultaten. 2007". www.lpz-um.nl/documents/lpz/lpz_rapport_2007_secured.pdf. Date of consultation: 27 October 2008.

xiv. De Ridder, D. et al., "The nutritional status of elderly in Belgian home nursing care (NAME-Study)", in Bayens, J.P. (ed.), *Gerontology and Geriatrie 1998. Proceedings of the 21st winter meeting*, Garant Leuven/Apeldoorn, Oostende, 2002, pp. 46-47, ISBN 90-441-1246-5.

xv. Smoliner, C. et al., "Effects of food fortification on nutritional and functional status in frail elderly nursing home residents at risk of malnutrition", *Nutrition*, 24 (11-12), pp. 1139-1144, published electronically ahead of print, 11 September 2008.

xvi. Locher, J.L. et al., "A multidimensional approach to understanding undereating in homebound older adults: the importance of social factors", *Gerontologist*, 48 (2), 2008, pp. 223-234.

xvii. Nijs, K. et al., "Effect of family style meals on quality of life, physical performance, and body weight of nursing home residents: cluster randomised controlled trial", *BMJ*, 332, 2006, pp. 1180-1184.

xviii. Haute Authorité de Santé, "Clinical Practice Guidelines. Nutritional support strategy for protein-energy malnutrition in the elderly", April 2007. www.has-sante.fr/portail/upload/docs/application/pdf/malnutrition_elderly_guidelines.pdf. Date of consultation: 27 October 2008.

xix. Schols, J., presentation at the Forum on Undernutrition in Care Homes and Home Care, November 2007.

xx. Lesourd, B. et al., "Comment favoriser la prise alimentaire des sujets âgés ?", *Nutr Clin Metabl,* 15, 2001, pp. 177-188.

xxi. Goode, H.F., Burns, E. and Walker, B.E., "Vitamin C depletion and pressure sores in elderly patients with femoral neck fracture", *BMJ (Clin Res Ed)*, 305, 1992, pp. 925-927.

xxii. Pierron, R.L., Perry, 3rd H.M., Grossberg, G., Morley, J.E., Mahon, G. and Stewart, T., "The aging hip", St. Louis University Geriatric Grand Rounds, *J Am Geriatr Soc*, 38, 1990, pp. 1339-1352.

xxiii. Chapuy, M.C., Pamphile, R., Paris, E., Kempf, C., Schlichting, M., Arnaud, S. et al., "Combined calcium and vitamin D3 supplementation in elderly women: confirmation of reversal of secondary hyperparathyroidism and hip fracture risk: the Decalyos II study", *Osteoporos Int*, 13, 2002, pp. 257-264.

xxiv. Chapuy, M.C., Schott, A.M., Garnero, P., Hans, D., Delmas, P.D. and Meunier, P.J., "Healthy elderly French women living at home have secondary hyperparathyroidism and high bone turnover in winter", EPIDOS Study Group, *Curr Opin Clin Nutr Metab Care*, 81, 1996, pp. 1129-1133.

xxv. Anderson, M.D., Collins, G., Davis, G., Bivins and B.A., "Malnutrition and length of stay: a relationship?", *Henry Ford Hosp Med J*, 59, 1985, pp. 477-483.

xxvi. UK health data 2006 from the presentation by Elia, M., at the Forum on Undernutrition in Care Homes and Home Care, November 2007.

xxvii. Elia, M., Stratton, R., Russell, C., Green, C. and Pang, F., "The cost of disease-related malnutrition in the UK and economic considerations for the use of oral nutritional supplements (ONS) in adults", BAPEN, Redditch, 2005.

xxviii. Elia, M. et al., "A cost-utility analysis in patients receiving enteral tube feeding at home and in nursing homes", *Clin Nutr*, 27 (3), 2008, pp. 416-423.

xxix. House of Commons Health Committee, "Obesity. Third report of session 2003-04. Volume 1", 27 May 2004. www.publications.parliament.uk/pa/cm200304 /cmselect/cmhealth/23/23.pdf. Date of consultation: 27 October 2008.

xxx. Ockenga, J. et al., "Nutritional assessment and management in hospitalised patients: implication for DRG-based reimbursement and health care quality", Clin Nutr, 24 (6), 2005, pp. 913-919.

xxxi. Pepersack, T. on behalf of the College for Geriatrics, "Outcomes of continuous process improvement of nutritional care program among geriatric units", *J Gerontol A Biol Sci Med Sci*, 60, 2005, pp. 787-792.

xxxii. Guigoz, Y., Vellas, B. and Garry, P.J., "Mini nutritional assessment: a practical assessment tool for grading the nutritional state of elderly patients", *Facts Res Gerontol*, Suppl. 2, 1994, pp. 15-59. www.mna-elderly.com. Date of consultation: 27 October 2008.

xxxiii. Wikby, K. et al., "The two-step Mini Nutritional Assessment procedure in community resident homes", J Clin Nurs, 17 (9), 2008, pp. 1211-1218, published electronically ahead of print, 11 February 2008.

xxxiv. MUST: Malnutrition Universal Screening Tool, BAPEN Nutrition Advisory Group. www.bapen.org.uk/must_tool.html. Date of consultation: 27 October 2008.

xxxv. Detsky, A.S., Mclaughin, J.R. and Baker, J.P., "What is subjective global assessment of nutritional status?", *JPEN*, 11 (8), 1987.

xxxvi. Milne, A.C., Potter, J. and Avenell, A., "Protein and energy supplementation in elderly people at risk from malnutrition", *The Cochrane Database of Systematic Reviews 2005*, Issue 1, Art. No: CD003288.pub2. doi:10.1002/14651858. CD003288.pub2.

xxxvii. Dupertuis, Y. et al., "Food intake in 1 707 hospitalised patients: a prospective comprehensive hospital survey", *Clin Nutr*, (22) 2, 2003, pp. 115-123.

xxxviii. Elia, M. et al., "Geographical inequalities in nutrient status and risk of malnutrition among English people aged 65 years and older", *Nutrition*, 21 (11-12), 2005, pp. 1100-1006.

xxxix. Weeks, L.E., "Participation in physical activity: influences reported by seniors in the community and in long-term care facilities", *J Gerontol Nurs*, 34 (7), 2008, pp. 36-43.

xl. Haute Autorité de Santé, "Quick reference guide. Nutritional support strategy for protein-energy malnutrition in the elderly", Haute Autorité de Santé, Service communication, Saint-Denis La Plaine; 2007. www.has-sante.fr/portail/upload/docs/application/pdf/malnutrition_elderly_quick_ref_guide.pdf. Date of consultation: 27 October 2008.

xli. www.mangerbouger.fr/IMG/pdf/PNNS2-Complet.pdf. Date of consultation: 27 October 2008.

xlii. Di Giulio, P. et al., "Dying with advanced dementia in long-term care geriatric institutions: a retrospective study", *J Palliat Med*, 11 (7), 2008, pp. 1023-1028.

xliii. www.alzheimers.org.uk. Date of consultation: 27 October 2008.

xliv. Shapiro, D.S. and Friedmann, R., "To feed or not to feed the terminal demented patient: is there any question?", IMAJ, 8, 2006, pp. 507–508.

xlv. Summersall, J. and Wight, S., "When it's difficult to swallow: the role of the speech therapist", in Hughes, J.C. (ed.), *Palliative Care in Severe Dementia*, Quay Books, 2006, pp. 105-113.

xlvi. www.ncpc.org.uk. Date of consultation: 27 October 2008.

xlvii. Beck, A.M. et al., "Food and nutritional care in hospitals: how to prevent undernutrition – Report and guidelines from the Council of Europe", *Clinical Nutrition*, 20 (5), pp. 455-460.

xlviii. Brown, L.E. et al., "Nutritional care in care homes: experiences and attitudes of care home staff", *J Hum Nutr Diet*, 15, 21 (4), 2008, p. 383.

xlix. Lindorff-Larsen, K. et al., "Management and perception of hospital undernutrition – A positive change among Danish doctors and nurses", *Clinical Nutrition*, 26 (3), 2007, pp. 371-378.

l. Schindler, K., presentation at the Forum on Undernutrition in Care Homes and Home Care, November 2007. www.nutritionday.org.

li. www.nutritionday.org/uploads/media/Valentini_Ernaehrung2007_01.pdf. Date of consultation: 27 October 2008.

lii. Pirlich, M. et al., "The German hospital malnutrition study", *Clinical Nutrition*, 25 (4), pp. 563-572.

liii. Sloane, P.D., "Nutritional issues in long-term care", *J Am Med Dir Assoc*, 9 (7), 2008, pp. 476-485.

liv. Kondrup, J., Allison, S.P., Elia, M., Vellas, B. and Plauth, M., "ESPEN guidelines for nutrition screening 2002", *Clinical Nutrition*, 22, 2003, pp. 415-421.

lv. Simmons, S.F., "Prevention of unintentional weight loss in nursing home residents: a controlled trial of feeding assistance", *J Am Geriatr Soc*, 56 (8), 2008, pp. 1466-1473.

lvi. www.vilans.nl, www.zorgvoorbeter.nl. Date of consultation: 27 October 2008.

lvii. Beck, A.M. et al., "Multifaceted nutritional intervention among nursing-home residents has a positive influence on nutrition and function", *Nutrition*, 24 (11-12), 2008, pp. 1073-1080, published electronically ahead of print 30 June 2008.

lviii. Johnson, C.S., Adequacy of nutrient intake among elderly persons receiving home care", *J Nutr Elder*, 27 (1-2), 2008, pp. 65-82.

lix. www.snellerbeter.nl; www.zorgvoorbeter.nl. Date of consultation: 27 October 2008.

lx. "Les recommandations Canicule" from the Health Ministry services. www.sante.gouv.fr/canicule.

lxi. Kohl, O., Dusseldorf, Schubert Unternehmensgruppe, "Meals in home care: balance between quality and cost", presentation at the Forum on Undernutrition in Care Homes and Home Care, November 2007.

lxii. www.deutsche-seniorenliga.de/ini.php. Date of consultation: 27 October 2008.

lxiii. www.european-nutrition.org/files/pdf_pdf_43.pdf. Date of consultation: 27 October 2008.

lxiv. European Commission. White paper on a Strategy for Europe on Nutrition, Overweight and Obesity related health issues. COM(2007) 279 final. Brussels, 30.5.2007.

http://ec.europa.eu/health/ph_determinants/life_style/nutrition/documents/nutrition_wp_en.pdf

lxv. European Parliament. Resolution on 'Together for Health: A Strategic Approach for the EU 2008-2013'. 2008/2115(INI). 9 October 2008. http://www.europarl.europa.eu/sides/getDoc.do?pubRef=-//EP//TEXT+TA+P6-TA-2008-0477+0+DOC+XML+V0//EN&language=EN

Sales agents for publications of the Council of Europe
Agents de vente des publications du Conseil de l'Europe

BELGIUM/BELGIQUE
La Librairie Européenne -
The European Bookshop
Rue de l'Orme, 1
BE-1040 BRUXELLES
Tel.: +32 (0)2 231 04 35
Fax: +32 (0)2 735 08 60
E-mail: order@libeurop.be
http://www.libeurop.be

Jean De Lannoy/DL Services
Avenue du Roi 202 Koningslaan
BE-1190 BRUXELLES
Tel.: +32 (0)2 538 43 08
Fax: +32 (0)2 538 08 41
E-mail: jean.de.lannoy@dl-servi.com
http://www.jean-de-lannoy.be

BOSNIA AND HERZEGOVINA/ BOSNIE-HERZÉGOVINE
Robert's Plus d.o.o.
Marka Maruliça 2/V
BA-71000, SARAJEVO
Tel.: + 387 33 640 818
Fax: + 387 33 640 818
E-mail: robertsplus@bih.net.ba

CANADA
Renouf Publishing Co. Ltd.
1-5369 Canotek Road
CA-OTTAWA, Ontario K1J 9J3
Tel.: +1 613 745 2665
Fax: +1 613 745 7660
Toll-Free Tel.: (866) 767-6766
E-mail: order.dept@renoufbooks.com
http://www.renoufbooks.com

CROATIA/CROATIE
Robert's Plus d.o.o.
Marasoviçeva 67
HR-21000, SPLIT
Tel.: + 385 21 315 800, 801, 802, 803
Fax: + 385 21 315 804
E-mail: robertsplus@robertsplus.hr

CZECH REPUBLIC/ RÉPUBLIQUE TCHÈQUE
Suweco CZ, s.r.o.
Klecakova 347
CZ-180 21 PRAHA 9
Tel.: +420 2 424 59 204
Fax: +420 2 848 21 646
E-mail: import@suweco.cz
http://www.suweco.cz

DENMARK/DANEMARK
GAD
Vimmelskaftet 32
DK-1161 KØBENHAVN K
Tel.: +45 77 66 60 00
Fax: +45 77 66 60 01
E-mail: gad@gad.dk
http://www.gad.dk

FINLAND/FINLANDE
Akateeminen Kirjakauppa
PO Box 128
Keskuskatu 1
FI-00100 HELSINKI
Tel.: +358 (0)9 121 4430
Fax: +358 (0)9 121 4242
E-mail: akatilaus@akateeminen.com
http://www.akateeminen.com

FRANCE
La Documentation française
(diffusion/distribution France entière)
124, rue Henri Barbusse
FR-93308 AUBERVILLIERS CEDEX
Tél.: +33 (0)1 40 15 70 00
Fax: +33 (0)1 40 15 68 00
E-mail: commande@ladocumentationfrancaise.fr
http://www.ladocumentationfrancaise.fr

Librairie Kléber
1 rue des Francs Bourgeois
FR-67000 STRASBOURG
Tel.: +33 (0)3 88 15 78 88
Fax: +33 (0)3 88 15 78 80
E-mail: librairie-kleber@coe.int
http://www.librairie-kleber.com

GERMANY/ALLEMAGNE AUSTRIA/AUTRICHE
UNO Verlag GmbH
August-Bebel-Allee 6
DE-53175 BONN
Tel.: +49 (0)228 94 90 20
Fax: +49 (0)228 94 90 222
E-mail: bestellung@uno-verlag.de
http://www.uno-verlag.de

GREECE/GRÈCE
Librairie Kauffmann s.a.
Stadiou 28
GR-105 64 ATHINAI
Tel.: +30 210 32 55 321
Fax.: +30 210 32 30 320
E-mail: ord@otenet.gr
http://www.kauffmann.gr

HUNGARY/HONGRIE
Euro Info Service
Pannónia u. 58.
PF. 1039
HU-1136 BUDAPEST
Tel.: +36 1 329 2170
Fax: +36 1 349 2053
E-mail: euroinfo@euroinfo.hu
http://www.euroinfo.hu

ITALY/ITALIE
Licosa SpA
Via Duca di Calabria, 1/1
IT-50125 FIRENZE
Tel.: +39 0556 483215
Fax: +39 0556 41257
E-mail: licosa@licosa.com
http://www.licosa.com

MEXICO/MEXIQUE
Mundi-Prensa México, S.A. De C.V.
Río Pánuco, 141 Delegacíon Cuauhtémoc
MX-06500 MÉXICO, D.F.
Tel.: +52 (01)55 55 33 56 58
Fax: +52 (01)55 55 14 67 99
E-mail: mundiprensa@mundiprensa.com.mx
http://www.mundiprensa.com.mx

NETHERLANDS/PAYS-BAS
Roodveldt Import BV
Nieuwe Hemweg 50
NE-1013 CX AMSTERDAM
Tel.: + 31 20 622 8035
Fax.: + 31 20 625 5493
Website: www.publidis.org
Email: orders@publidis.org

NORWAY/NORVÈGE
Akademika
Postboks 84 Blindern
NO-0314 OSLO
Tel.: +47 2 218 8100
Fax: +47 2 218 8103
E-mail: support@akademika.no
http://www.akademika.no

POLAND/POLOGNE
Ars Polona JSC
25 Obroncow Street
PL-03-933 WARSZAWA
Tel.: +48 (0)22 509 86 00
Fax: +48 (0)22 509 86 10
E-mail: arspolona@arspolona.com.pl
http://www.arspolona.com.pl

PORTUGAL
Livraria Portugal
(Dias & Andrade, Lda.)
Rua do Carmo, 70
PT-1200-094 LISBOA
Tel.: +351 21 347 42 82 / 85
Fax: +351 21 347 02 64
E-mail: info@livrariaportugal.pt
http://www.livrariaportugal.pt

RUSSIAN FEDERATION/ FÉDÉRATION DE RUSSIE
Ves Mir
17b, Butlerova ul.
RU-101000 MOSCOW
Tel.: +7 495 739 0971
Fax: +7 495 739 0971
E-mail: orders@vesmirbooks.ru
http://www.vesmirbooks.ru

SPAIN/ESPAGNE
Mundi-Prensa Libros, s.a.
Castelló, 37
ES-28001 MADRID
Tel.: +34 914 36 37 00
Fax: +34 915 75 39 98
E-mail: libreria@mundiprensa.es
http://www.mundiprensa.com

SWITZERLAND/SUISSE
Planetis Sàrl
16 chemin des pins
CH-1273 ARZIER
Tel.: +41 22 366 51 77
Fax: +41 22 366 51 78
E-mail: info@planetis.ch

UNITED KINGDOM/ROYAUME-UNI
The Stationery Office Ltd
PO Box 29
GB-NORWICH NR3 1GN
Tel.: +44 (0)870 600 5522
Fax: +44 (0)870 600 5533
E-mail: book.enquiries@tso.co.uk
http://www.tsoshop.co.uk

UNITED STATES and CANADA/ ÉTATS-UNIS et CANADA
Manhattan Publishing Company
468 Albany Post Road
US-CROTON-ON-HUDSON, NY 10520
Tel.: +1 914 271 5194
Fax: +1 914 271 5856
E-mail: Info@manhattanpublishing.com
http://www.manhattanpublishing.com

Council of Europe Publishing/Editions du Conseil de l'Europe
FR-67075 STRASBOURG Cedex
Tel.: +33 (0)3 88 41 25 81 – Fax: +33 (0)3 88 41 39 10 – E-mail: publishing@coe.int – Website: http://book.coe.int